Professor John Hunter is a Consultant Physician at Addenbrooke's Hospital, Cambridge, a visiting Professor of Medicine at the University of Cranfield and a recognised authority on diseases of the gut including Irritable Bowel Syndrome, Crohn's Disease and Colitis. He has contributed over a hundred research papers to major medical journals including *The Lancet*, *Nature* and *The British Medical Journal* and is the author of *Solve Your Food Intolerance*.

IRRITABLE BOWEL SOLUTIONS

The essential guide to
Irritable Bowel Syndrome,
its causes and treatments

Professor John Hunter
MA, MD, FRCP, AGAF

Vermilion
LONDON

7 9 10 8 6

Published in 2007 by Vermilion, an imprint of Ebury Publishing

A Random House Group Company

The Random House Group Limited Reg. No. 954009

Addresses for companies within the Random House Group can be found at
www.rbooks.co.uk

A CIP catalogue record for this book is available from the British Library

The Random House Group Limited supports The Forest Stewardship Council
(FSC), the leading international forest certification organisation. All our titles
that are printed on Greenpeace approved FSC certified paper carry the FSC logo.
Our paper procurement policy can be found at
www.rbooks.co.uk/environment

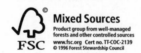

To buy books by your favourite authors and register for offers visit
www.rbooks.co.uk

Printed and bound in Great Britain by CPI Mackays, Chatham ME5 8TD

ISBN 9780091917067

Contents

Acknowledgements

The research on which this book is based was performed in the Gastroenterology Research Unit, Addenbrooke's Hospital, Cambridge, between 1982 and the present day. I acknowledge with grateful thanks the invaluable contributions made by many of my colleagues in that department over the years, especially those doctors who were brave enough to write MDs on Irritable Bowel Syndrome, including Virginia Alun Jones, Tim King and Keith Dear and those who completed PhDs in the field, whether at Cambridge or Cranfield – Valerie Sparkes, Jennifer Madden and Maria Pilar Montoya de Bilbao. I am also grateful for invaluable discussions with other medical colleagues in Cambridge over the years, particularly Marinos Elia, John Cummings, Sean Kelly, Steve Middleton, John Crampton and Sybil Birtwhistle.

Particular thanks must go to my dietitians beginning with Liz Workman, followed by Alex Riordan, Sharon Borland, Sally Naylor, Jenny Woolner, Jo Cotterell, Gillian Kirby, Tracy Parker, Monina Mullen, Eoghan Brennan and Vicky Chudleigh. Their patience and skill in developing the nutritional management of IBS and Crohn's disease can never be overestimated!

Dr Claude Lum introduced me to the clinical importance of chronic hyperventilation and for many years my patients with this problem were treated by Ann Copping whose care transformed many lives. Other physiotherapists working with me on musculo-skeletal problems in particular included Ros Brown and Anne-Marie Melloy. Our nurses have been deeply involved in the project particularly Quita Bartlett, Lynette Byatt, Allison Nightingale, Fiona Jorgenssen, Lizzie Dimmock and Mo Wiesner.

I am particularly grateful to Maria Shorthouse, whose technical skills were such that she could set up any assay which from time we thought might be necessary, and which enabled a small laboratory in Cambridge to punch well above its weight.

Over the years the activities of the Gastroenterology Research Unit were co-ordinated and its finances balanced by our managers, Alison Lee and later Sue Tarry, for whose help I shall always be extremely grateful.

My particular thanks are due to those colleagues who helped me by reading chapters of the book which were in their special domains, and for their wise and helpful suggestions. These included Ann Copping, Lynette Byatt, Ann-Marie Melloy, Sally Naylor and Peter Milton. Any mistakes, however, are mine, and not theirs!

My editor at Vermilion, Imogen Fortes, has been a model of diplomacy and charm. Finally, I must thank Sarah Basser for typing the manuscript and for her unfailing good temper and good humour and my wife Maureen who, with the rest of my family, has unfailingly supported me through long years of exploring the intricacies of IBS.

Introduction to IBS

ARE YOU CONFIDENT THAT YOUR PROBLEM IS IBS?

Irritable bowel syndrome (IBS) is a disorder involving the intestines (or bowels), especially the large bowel (or colon). You must be quite certain that IBS is indeed the cause of your symptoms. Diarrhoea, constipation, bloating and abdominal pain are symptoms that occur very frequently, and although IBS may be one of the most common causes of such symptoms in the developed world, there are many other possibilities. Nothing can be more tragic than the patient who, after trying for several months to control 'IBS', is found to have bowel cancer – possibly too late for successful treatment. The guidelines in this book are meant for patients who have been properly investigated by their doctors and where the diagnosis of IBS is soundly based.

If you have not been to see your doctor to check out your symptoms, do so straight away.

The following medical checks are the ones I recommend for my own patients to rule out more dangerous conditions:

BLOOD TESTS	STOOL TESTS
Full blood count Kidney function test Liver function test Thyroid function test Calcium and phosphorus levels Antibodies for coeliac disease Tests for inflammation – C-reactive protein or ESR	Examination of faeces for disease-causing (pathogenic) bacteria and parasites
In patients over 45 years of age, it is also important to examine the large bowel, either by x-ray or colonoscopy, to exclude cancer.	

THE OLD APPROACH TO IBS

In the past, many doctors believed that IBS was psycho-somatic – that is, caused by psychological upsets that lead to symptoms in the gut. This was because no signs of disease could be found in the bowel that might account for the pain. There are undoubtedly psychological factors involved. Anxiety, depression, panic and agoraphobia are all common in IBS patients, particularly those who are seen in hospital. The importance of anxiety in IBS is discussed in Chapter 7. Unfortunately, the belief that IBS is largely 'all in the mind' meant that it was dismissed by many as a minor problem – or even worse, an amusing one. Just the mention of 'IBS' was often sufficient to raise a smile at medical meetings. When pressure was mounting to dismiss Iain Duncan Smith as leader of the Conservative Party in Britain a few years ago, his opponents started to refer to him as 'IDS'. This sounded close enough to 'IBS' to make him appear a lightweight!

However, our experience at Addenbrooke's Hospital in Cambridge has shown that in only 20 per cent of cases is IBS produced by anxiety. Other research has shown that patients who are assessed shortly after their IBS symptoms occur show little if any psychological difference from healthy people. On the other hand, the many patients who have struggled with IBS for five years or more, with little if any relief, are frequently found, hardly surprisingly, to suffer from anxiety and depression – but this is the effect of the disease, not its cause.

THE IMPACT OF IBS

Because no serious disease can be discovered underlying IBS symptoms, it's often assumed that the problem is trivial. This is far from true. IBS is not a dangerous condition in that it does not lead on to the development of cancer or colitis (inflammation of the colon). Probably the only bowel disease that can be linked with IBS is diverticulosis (see page 186) which is, in any case, a common condition in the western world that becomes more likely from the age of 40 onwards, affecting more than half the population over the age of 80. From this it can be seen that the outlook for IBS sufferers is good – yet its effects may be devastating.

The abdominal pain of IBS may be very severe. One woman told me that she felt the pain of IBS was worse than childbirth. It's frequently bad enough to cause patients to have to leave the dinner table and retreat to an early bed. Urgent diarrhoea may mean that patients are terrified of being 'taken short' when out and about, for example when riding on a bus or underground train. Many have told me they know the exact locations of every public lavatory in the towns they visit regularly for shopping or entertainment and that they plan their routes to and from work meticulously so that they are always within easy reach of a loo!

Bowel symptoms always have the potential to cause great embarrassment, but in IBS this sort of problem can continue indefinitely, often with no apparent relief in sight, making sufferers' lives a misery. Patients with IBS do sometimes die because of the condition – they commit suicide.

Certainly IBS is not a minor problem. It is easily the commonest reason for referral to gastroenterology (disorders of the gut) services across the developed world. When patients with IBS are assessed for their quality of life it is found that, in terms of both social effects and their emotional state, IBS symptoms are comparable to (and sometimes worse than) symptoms of diseases such as depression, diabetes and high blood pressure. The annual direct costs of IBS in the UK have been estimated at over £46 million – and that was in 1998. In the USA it was even more at $1.6 billion (around £800 million).

HOW TO USE THIS BOOK

In general, this book will teach you how to control your irritable bowel syndrome but it has several specific functions:

1. To reassure you that sufferers from IBS are not 'wimps'. You simply have a medical problem for which help is available.

2. To provide a way of sorting out the abnormality that causes **your** IBS.

3. To offer advice on keeping your gut healthy afterwards.

4. To offer guidance on some of the misleading claims made by alternative practitioners that may confuse you.

It may contain more medical and scientific facts than you believe you require. That is for a reason, because knowledge is power. The more you understand about what is upsetting your gut, the better able you are to live with it and control it.

Knowledge allows you to make the best use of your own local medical resources. Your doctor is vital. Use him or her to best advantage. The information given in the book will ensure that your doctor takes your approach to your IBS seriously. You will be able to discuss problems with your consultant or GP on a more equal footing, so that your questions and anxieties cannot be brushed off lightly.

THE WAY FORWARD

If you have IBS, this book offers a way forward. There are six steps:

1. Check with your doctor that you do indeed suffer from IBS. Ask your doctor if you may stop any medication which might influence the symptoms which you suffer, such as laxatives or anti-diarrhoeals (but never stop medication without checking with your doctor first).

2. Study your symptoms for 10–14 days, making an accurate record as described in Chapters 2 and 3.
3. Calculate how long it takes for the food you

consume to pass out of your body. This is known as your 'whole gut transit time' or WGTT. (See page 25.)

4. Complete the questionnaire in Chapter 3 and make a note of the types of IBS for which you score positive.

5. Read the relevant chapter, outlining the treatment suggested for your type of IBS, and follow the advice provided. If you are positive for more than one, read Chapter 4 to see which type you should attack first.

6. Read Chapters 12 and 13 to help you continue to keep your bowel symptoms under control in the future.

Finally, each chapter ends with a short summary to remind you of the key points and to help you find them again later. Good luck!

CHAPTER 1

Why is There Confusion Over IBS?

The diagnosis of IBS depends on a discussion of the symptoms with your doctor – while also excluding any other causes for them. There is no characteristic symptom pattern that confirms IBS. The diagnosis depends entirely on the information the patient gives to the doctor regarding his or her symptoms and any other relevant details – known as a medical 'history'.

Even then, the diagnosis of IBS is not straightforward. This is because there is no single test that clearly confirms it. For many doctors, IBS just means any case of abdominal pain for which no cause can be discovered. The doctors may have listened to the patient's history, performed an examination, analysed the blood, checked the stools (faeces), and tested the urine, but all have proven completely normal.

Endoscopy (internal examination using a viewing device) to look at the stomach or large bowel, or x-rays such as barium enemas, may have been performed, but no abnormality has been discovered. After going through all this, the poor old patient is expected to be grateful that a wide range of diseases, in particular the dreaded cancer of the colon, has been excluded. Told that her symptoms are not caused by anything nasty, the patient is expected to smile and forget all about it. 'You'll just have to live with it, Mrs Smith!'

The reason that IBS has proved so confusing is that the lack of a specific test means that quite different disorders may be grouped together under the same name. When a disease, such as tuberculosis (TB), is well understood, it may be confidently diagnosed by isolating its cause – a bacterium (*Mycobacterium tuberculosis*). Whatever symptoms TB may cause – and it produces many, as it may affect different parts of the body – it makes no difference to the diagnosis. A person with TB may have a dreadful cough or severe pain the back, but the diagnosis is still the same.

When the cause of a condition is not well understood, doctors cannot make a precise diagnosis and must rely on symptoms alone. This is true, for example, of chronic fatigue syndrome (sometimes called ME, or 'yuppie flu') or of psychiatric disorders, such as depression. Conditions that produce the same sort of symptoms tend to be lumped together, but because they are classified by symptoms rather than by a true understanding of the cause, they are given the label of 'syndrome'.

Until research reveals what is going on behind the symptoms, there is always the risk that very different problems may be lumped together under the same heading. So it is with IBS. It merely means a condition in which abdominal pain occurs over quite a long period, and is associated with an irregular bowel habit. Because such symptoms occur with no discernible cause, it is called irritable bowel *syndrome*.

Attempts have been made to define the symptoms of IBS in such a way that comparable patients are enrolled for research into its cause, and not a mish-mash of wildly different cases. The 'Rome II Criteria', developed by a group of medical specialists at a meeting in Rome, are now widely used for this purpose. The Rome Criteria, however, cannot even reliably distinguish between IBS and say, Crohn's disease, cancer or colitis. Nor do they provide a basis on which doctors can confidently suggest a treatment. They merely make sure the right sorts of IBS patients go into clinical trials.

The Rome Criteria are shown in full below. The IBS symptoms are followed by a list of symptoms that are not found in IBS and so will suggest to the doctor that there may be a different, and potentially more dangerous, condition. They are known as 'red flag' symptoms.

THE ROME II CRITERIA 1999

For at least **12** weeks or more (not necessarily consecutive), in the preceding 12 months, the sufferer will have abdominal discomfort or pain with **two** out of the following three features:

➤ Relieved by defecation and/or
➤ Onset associated with a change in the frequency of stool and/or
➤ Onset associated with a change in the form/appearance of stool.

Other features (part of the previous and more complex Rome I criteria) that are often present, include:

➤ Abnormal stool frequency
➤ Abnormal stool form
➤ Abnormal passage of stool (straining, urgency or feeling of incomplete evacuation)
➤ Passage of mucus
➤ Bloating or feeling of abdominal distension.

POTENTIAL IBS SYMPTOMS

Put more simply, the primary symptom is discomfort and pain in the abdomen that comes and goes over a one-year period but lasts – in total – at least three months. Pain is relieved by defecation and associated with diarrhoea and/or constipation. Patients with IBS may alternate between diarrhoea and constipation, which means that they pass several stools one day and nothing at all on the next couple of days.

Patients may have to rush to the lavatory, or strain when they are on the lavatory, or feel they haven't finished and yet cannot pass any more stools. They may pass mucus with their stools, and feel that their abdomen is swollen and bloated. I look at these symptoms in more detail in the next chapter. As we shall see, however, although diarrhoea and/or constipation may be major factors in IBS, their relative importance may not always be obvious.

'RED FLAG' SYMPTOMS

The following symptoms are NOT seen in IBS and must always be investigated further:

➤ Weight loss.
➤ Blood in the stools.
➤ Abdominal pain or diarrhoea during the night.
➤ Anaemia.
➤ Fever.

As you can see from the wide range of symptoms, IBS is not one distinct condition – but several. When a number of different conditions are included under the same diagnosis, and there is no objective test that can confirm the condition, it is hardly surprising that doctors become confused. Wildly inappropriate treatments may be recommended, and many doctors come to feel that it is no use offering any treatment at all. I believe, however, that knowledge of the symptoms of IBS has now reached the stage where patients may be reliably classified in such a way that sensible treatments may be recommended.

SUMMARY

➤ IBS symptoms are not 'all in the mind' and can be treated.

➤ IBS is not dangerous but can have a serious impact on your quality of life.

➤ IBS involves pain in the abdomen for which no other cause can be found.

➤ There may be diarrhoea and/or constipation, and abdominal bloating.

➤ If you have these symptoms, see your doctor for advice and to rule out more dangerous conditions.

CHAPTER 2

What are the Symptoms of IBS?

As the diagnosis and treatment of IBS are based on symptoms it is crucial that a patient describes them correctly. However, IBS is a very common complaint and the symptoms could be the result of a wide range of different problems. Medical terms such as diarrhoea and constipation are nowadays all used freely in general conversation. However, doctor and patient may interpret the same word quite differently.

A good example of this is the use of the term 'chronic' to describe symptoms. Doctors use it to describe symptoms that are long-lasting and persistent. It helps distinguish chronic symptoms from symptoms that occur suddenly, or that started only recently, or are short-lived, which are known as 'acute'. But many patients believe chronic pain to be one that is particularly severe and unpleasant, whether it lasts for five minutes or five months. 'When the pain comes on, doctor, it's really chronic.'

When such terms are misunderstood it can lead to problems, especially when diagnosis depends on the correct interpretation of symptoms – as is the case with IBS. This was clearly shown in a study of a group of patients diagnosed with IBS in which over half said their main symptom was diarrhoea. When their stools were weighed, however, it was found that they were well within the normal range. Yet stools are rarely weighed in routine medical practice, and so it is likely these patients would, in the usual course of events, have been given medicines to stop diarrhoea – which would have proved ineffective. If the patient doesn't give the doctor a clear description of what's going on, the wrong treatment may very likely be suggested.

In this chapter, I'm going to discuss the common symptoms of IBS in detail so that you have a better idea of how your bowels are working. You can then describe the problem accurately so that you and your doctor are on the same wavelength.

ABDOMINAL PAIN

As we saw in Chapter 1, abdominal pain is the prime symptom of IBS and so is the first and most important one to consider. Indeed, if there is no pain, it is not strictly possible to make a diagnosis of IBS. Some people include diarrhoea that is not painful but with no apparent cause as a form of IBS, but that is probably a separate condition. Nevertheless, it often responds successfully to one of the treatments I recommend in this book – an exclusion diet – as described in Chapter 5.

IBS pain has been studied by placing balloons in various places inside the gut of IBS patients and non-sufferers. The balloon is inflated until it becomes painful, and the pressure inside the balloon at this moment is measured. It has been found that, in IBS patients, the pain is felt at a much lower pressure than in non-sufferers. This is called 'visceral hypersensitivity', which simply means the gut is more sensitive to pain in IBS – hardly surprising! Despite this, the gut appears to be quite healthy in IBS.

This has led to suggestions that the cause of the pain is not in the gut at all, but in the brain. Nerve signals are continuously passing from gut to brain. In normal individuals, however, these do not produce any discomfort. Perhaps in IBS, the stresses and strains of modern life lead to increased sensitivity in the brain itself, so signals that in normal individuals cause no trouble lead to pain in IBS patients?

An alternative explanation may be that there are simply more signals from the gut. Perhaps because of abnormal fermentation (malfermentation – see page 53), or constipation, the wall of the bowel might be stiffer, or more sensitive than would usually be the case, leading to an increase in nerve signals to the brain. This latter theory has yet to be confirmed by research.

Many patients find it quite frustrating when their doctor can't seem to determine the source of their abdominal pain. If patients have a pain in a finger they can point to it and the doctor knows full well where the trouble lies. When patients have a pain in their belly, they can point to the area affected and will again expect their doctor to know exactly where the pain is coming from and what is causing it.

Unfortunately, pain from the abdominal organs is much more difficult to identify than pain in the limbs. Nerves pass from the abdominal organs to the spinal cord and these connect to other nerves that relay information up to the brain. Here, yet a third type of nerve sends information to the conscious part of the brain. However, there are relatively few nerves passing from the abdominal organs to the spinal cord and one nerve may originate from several sites. Even more importantly, a single nerve entering the spinal cord may connect with several other nerves going up towards the brain. This makes it very difficult to be precise about exactly where the pain is coming from.

The situation is further complicated because if a nerve from the gut enters the spine at the same level as a nerve supplying muscles and joints, the pain may falsely seem to come from those muscles and joints. This is called 'referred pain' because it has been *referred* from one part of the body to another.

The gallbladder, for example, lies under the lower ribs on the right, and that is where patients may expect to feel gallbladder pain. 'Classical' gallbladder pain, however, is felt in the middle of the upper abdomen and often spreads to the shoulder or right shoulder blade. It is only when the gallbladder becomes inflamed (acute cholecystitis) and the inflammation spreads to surrounding tissues that pain is felt on the right hand side of the upper abdomen. Heart disease, gallstones, oesophagitis and IBS may all cause pain behind the breastbone. It's therefore important to know where the pain may spread.

The doctor also needs to know when the pain comes on, not only the time of day, but also whether it follows activities such as meals or physical exertion. It is crucial to discover any factors that may make the pain better or worse, such as heavier breathing, or a change in posture. Stomach pains may be relieved by eating or by antacid medicines. Both reduce stomach acid.

Bowel pain tends to improve after passing wind or a stool as this reduces the pressure in the bowel (like letting down a balloon). Finally, it also helps to know if the pain is accompanied by any other symptoms. Pain accompanied by blood in the urine, for example, is more likely to be due to kidney disease.

Other studies have shown that in patients with IBS – unlike in non-sufferers – the whole gut is a potential source of pain and in any individual patient, more than one site may be involved. In IBS it is therefore more important to consider the nature of the pain rather than its site.

A good doctor will of course ask all these questions when trying to get to the root of a patient's pain. However, the patient who, as well as being unwell, is often nervous at meeting a strange new doctor, may not have had the opportunity to consider the correct answer to an unexpected question that is suddenly thrust upon him or her. Below we list the important factors that may involve symptoms of IBS so that you may think about these things before you see your doctor and thus provide accurate answers.

PAIN	BOWELS
Where is the pain felt?	How many times do you pass stools each week?
Where does the pain spread to?	How many times do you pass stools each day?
When does the pain come on?	What is the typical appearance of your stools?
What makes the pain better? Can you do anything to relieve the pain?	Are there any regular variations in stool habit?
Does anything make the pain worse?	Do the stools contain any mucus or blood?

CHARACTERISTIC PAIN OF IBS

IBS pain usually occurs across the belly below the navel, but may arise anywhere in the abdomen. It is usually associated with bloating and often comes on after you start eating, which causes the gut to contract by a reflex (called the gastro-colic reflex). In women, it may be worse in the days leading up to a period. It is characteristically relieved by passing wind or a stool.

Although this description is typical IBS pain, always tell your doctor what **you** notice, and don't try to force your symptoms into the 'typical' mould! **Never** try to tell the doctor what you think he or she wants to hear – describe your symptoms simply and accurately, trying to think how the pain may be affected by all the different factors that we have mentioned.

There is often a change in the frequency or appearance of the stools, as well. As we shall see, the nature of such a change in the form of a stool is crucial in sorting out which form of IBS is responsible for the pain – and is of much more value than the nature of the pain itself.

BLOATING

Bloating is when the abdomen swells. There are five major causes of bloating – each beginning with the letter F: Fat, Foetus (i.e. pregnancy), Fluid, Faeces (i.e. constipation) and Flatus (wind). Only the last two are relevant to IBS, although female patients have often been referred to gastroenterologists with suspected IBS who in fact turn out to be pregnant! Pregnancy does, after all, produce various gastrointestinal symptoms. The presence of fluid in the abdomen (ascites) is a sign of important disease and is never caused by IBS.

Severe constipation may lead to a degree of abdominal distension that the doctor can feel when he examines the patient's abdomen. If constipation is the cause, this bloating will disappear after a bowel clearout. The main cause of abdominal bloating in IBS is gas. Our research has shown that the production of hydrogen gas in IBS is vastly increased (see Chapter 5).

CASE STUDY

Gas may produce remarkable abdominal distension. I once had a patient who kept three separate wardrobes. Being a busy, successful career woman she had to attend a number of business meals and was well aware that her distension became worse after eating. She would go along to a meal in one of the smaller outfits but take outfit three, the largest, with her. When the distension began to get so bad that she thought her buttons were going to burst, she would slip out to the loo and slip into something more comfortable! Fortunately, when her food intolerances had been sorted out, she was able to get by with a single set of clothes – the smallest.

Although bloating is very common in IBS, it's not a symptom of great value in distinguishing one type of IBS from another. An excess of gas in the bowel may be due to the fermentation of food residues by the bacteria that live in the large intestine (Chapter 5), or may arise from air swallowing, which is typically a symptom of anxiety (Chapter 7).

In practical terms, the best way to distinguish between the two is by the presence or absence of belching. When we swallow air, although some passes through the stomach into the bowel, a considerable amount passes back up the gullet (oesophagus), and in many patients is expelled by belching.

Gas produced by fermentation, however, cannot be belched up under normal circumstances. This would require a journey from the large bowel back to the stomach, along some 6 m (20 ft) of twisting, turning small intestine, swimming against the prevailing current.

Simply asking how often the patient belches may be enough to put the doctor on the right track.

DIARRHOEA

The formal definition of diarrhoea, in adults in the developed world, is of a daily stool output of more than 200 g. In practice, this usually means two or more loose stools each day. Considering how much fluid passes through the gut in a normal day, it's surprising diarrhoea is not more frequent. Some 10 litres (over 17 pints) of fluid enter the small intestine each day, by mouth and in secretions from the digestive glands. Three-quarters of this is reabsorbed in the small intestine and the rest in the large intestine, so that a normal stool volume is only about 200mls (1/5th litre).

Diarrhoea can occur by four gut mechanisms:

➤ Increased secretion of fluids.
➤ Reduced absorption of fluids.
➤ Chemicals that increase the flow of fluid into the bowel.
➤ Increased bowel motility (movement).

In IBS it seems likely that secretion may be increased by the over-production of hormone-like chemicals called prostaglandins and also by increased bowel motility. The most common over-all reason for diarrhoea is infection and this usually lasts less than a fortnight. Most people have no doubt at all when they are suffering from this sort of problem. In IBS, however, the definition of diarrhoea may be more problematic.

Some patients record that they have diarrhoea when they pass stools frequently, others when they pass stools that are loose. In practice, I ask patients who report that they have diarrhoea whether they mean that the stools are frequent or loose or both. Diarrhoea is usually associated with an urgent need to rush to the lavatory.

CASE STUDY

The difficulty in describing diarrhoea is illustrated by the case of one of my patients, a man who suffered from 'IBS' for over 20 years. He had visited various specialists up and down the country trying medications such as anti-depressants, hypnotism and all manner of diets, with absolutely no success. He considered that he had diarrhoea as he was passing seven to eight stools per day. They were associated with a most unpleasant lower abdominal and anal pain, which was so bad that he had had to give up work. He repeatedly took anti-diarrhoeal drugs such as codeine and loperamide without getting any better.

We admitted him to the hospital for further investigation and the nurses noted that his stools were in fact very small. We weighed them and he produced a mere 75 g in 24 hours. Clearly, this could not be diarrhoea and on questioning he admitted that his stools were usually like 'chipolatas'. Further investigation confirmed that he was suffering from constipation due to spasms in the muscles of the floor of the pelvis. He had had a very painful fissure in his anus. When he went to the lavatory to pass a motion he had developed the habit of contracting the muscles of the pelvic floor (see page 125) instead of relaxing them, to protect himself against the pain from the fissure as stools passed through his anus. Treating him with anti-diarrhoea drugs was making the problem worse. When his constipation was treated his symptoms rapidly subsided.

A further difficulty with diarrhoea in IBS is that it may be intermittent. Indeed, many descriptions of IBS stress the way that there may be alternating constipation and diarrhoea. Because diarrhoea is awkward, embarrassing and difficult to deal with, patients tend to complain most about that aspect of their bowel function, rather than on what happens to their stools in between the bouts of diarrhoea.

The nature of the stools in between the diarrhoea may be more important than what happens during the attack itself. Thus in Chapter 6 we discuss 'overload and overflow', where patients pass small hard stools for a week to 10 days at a time, but the bowel does not empty completely and the amount of residue builds up until there is sufficient to trigger a bout of overflow diarrhoea.

The diarrhoea is the dramatic event that demands treatment, but underlying it is a chronic degree of constipation that gets worse if, as frequently happens, the diarrhoea is treated with an anti-diarrhoea drug such as loperamide.

Some prescription drugs quite often produce diarrhoea (see below), including antibiotics and beta blockers. If you think your medication may be a factor in your symptoms, discuss it with your doctor. **However, never stop medical treatment without talking to your doctor first.**

DRUGS THAT MAY CAUSE DIARRHOEA

5-aminosalicylates, e.g. olsalazine, mesalazine
Antibiotics
Azathioprine
Beta blockers, e.g. propranolol, atenolol
Calcitonin

Colchicine
Drugs used for chemotherapy of cancer and other tumours
Gold, either by injection or by mouth (auranofin)
Iron preparations, e.g. ferrous sulphate
Methyldopa
Metformin
Magnesium salts used as either antacids or laxatives
Misoprostol
Non-steroidal anti-inflammatory drugs, e.g. mefenamic acid, indomethacin, diclofenac
Proton pump inhibitors, e.g. omeprazole, lansoprazole
Statins
Thyroxine

This list is not exhaustive, and if your symptoms begin or get worse after starting any drug you should discuss it with your doctor.

CONSTIPATION

Constipation is the reason for over 2.5 million visits to the doctor and millions of pounds are spent each year on laxatives. It is clearly a major medical problem and yet there is considerable disagreement between lay people and their doctors as to exactly what the term means.

To many, constipation means going to the lavatory infrequently. It is estimated that 98 per cent of the population have a stool frequency varying from three stools a week to three stools a day. Some doctors have suggested that a practical definition of constipation might be the passage of less than three stools each week.

However, the problem has become more complex because the simple definition of constipation as 'infrequent stools' has now been expanded to include difficulty in passing stools. This is a concept that is highly subjective and difficult to quantify – it may include straining to empty the bowel, the passage of lumpy or hard stools, the feeling that the bowel has not been completely emptied or that there is some sort of 'blockage' at the lower end of the bowel.

These various symptoms have been grouped together by the same group of doctors who classified IBS and are known as the Rome II Criteria for Constipation (see page 120 for full list). The essential difference between constipation and IBS is that simple constipation does not cause abdominal pain, whereas IBS, of course, does.

SYMPTOMS OF CONSTIPATION

Constipation is regarded as three bowel movements or fewer per week plus two or more of the following symptoms for at least 12 weeks (not necessarily consecutive) in the preceding 12 months in more than 25 per cent of bowel movements:

➤ Straining.
➤ Lumpy or hard stools.
➤ Sensation of incomplete evacuation (that is, you don't feel that you've finished).
➤ Sensation of anal/rectal blockage.
➤ Manually assisting bowel evacuation (that is, using the hands to help).

As you will see (Chapter 6), urgent diarrhoea may occur in some cases where there is underlying constipation, and treatment for such diarrhoea with anti-diarrhoea drugs only makes the underlying problem worse. Furthermore, some people have a bowel habit that would fulfil the criteria for constipation, yet would not consider for a moment that their bowels were in any way a problem.

In many cases of constipation, the loaded bowel can be felt when the abdomen is examined, but again this may occur in patients who have no worries about their bowels at all. Clearly, constipation is not a simple and straight-forward subject.

Scientifically, constipation may be evaluated in two ways – by measurement of the time it takes food to pass through the body – called the 'whole gut transit time' (WGTT), which should be less than three days (70 hours) – and by measuring the weight of the stool.

To determine the whole gut transit time, the patient is asked to swallow special markers that show up on x-rays. A known number of markers are swallowed each day and x-rays are taken at intervals to reveal their position in the intestine. From this the WGTT is calculated.

Faecal weight simply involves collecting the stools passed over a 24-hour period and weighing them. In Western Europe, the average daily stool weight is 150–200 g, but may be much less in constipated patients. The most reliable way of proving constipation scientif-ically is by WGTT, but neither technique is of much help for the ordinary person at home trying to work out whether or not he or she is truly constipated, so how can you detect it?

Fortunately, help is available. A group of physicians in Bristol, led by Dr Ken Heaton, have performed sterling work in the understanding of IBS. They discovered that the best guide was a change in the form of the stool. They asked 66 volunteers to keep a diary of the number of times they went to the lavatory and how the stool looked.

They repeated this after being given a laxative and then an anti-diarrhoea drug. Using this information, Dr Heaton's team developed the 'Bristol Stool Form Scale' (see below), which gives a valuable indication of the whole gut transit time – and hence whether or not the patient has constipation – based on the form of the stool.

BRISTOL STOOL FORM SCALE

➤ **Type 1**: Separate hard lumps like nuts.

➤ **Type 2**: Sausage-like but lumpy.

➤ **Type 3**: Sausage-like but with cracks in the surface.

➤ **Type 4**: Sausage- and snake-like, smooth and soft.

➤ **Type 5**: Soft blobs with clear cut edges.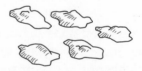

➤ **Type 6**: Fluffy pieces with ragged edges, a mushy stool.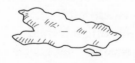

➤ **Type 7**: Watery with no solid pieces (entirely liquid).

Stools at the lumpy end of the scale are hard to pass and often require a lot of straining. Stools at the loose or liquid end of the spectrum can be too easy to pass – they may produce urgency and accidents. The ideal stools are Types 3 and 4, especially Type 4, as they are most likely to glide out without any fuss at all. They are also least likely to leave an annoying feeling that something has been left behind, which still remains to be passed (hence 'incomplete evacuation').

The average time for the passage of undigested food residues through the gut is:

➤ **Men:** just over two days (50 hours).
➤ **Women:** just under two and a half days (57 hours).

But it can range from less than a day (20 hours) to more than four days (100 hours). The undigested residue spends most of this time passing along the large intestine. The time taken changes from one day to the next. This is one reason why we do not produce the same sort of stool each day.

NAUSEA AND VOMITING

Nausea and vomiting do not occur very often in IBS. This may seem surprising, given the sensitive nature of the whole of the gut in IBS. In practice, nausea and vomiting are usually only seen in IBS caused by anxiety where air swallowing may distend the stomach, leading to nausea or – in more sensitive people – repeated vomiting. This is discussed in more detail in Chapter 7.

SYMPTOMS OUTSIDE THE GUT

There are, of course, many other symptoms reported by patients with IBS, ranging from tiredness or headache to frequent urination and aches in the joints. None of these, however tiresome they may be, are of importance in the diagnosis of IBS, nor in working out the best way to treat it. All patients with IBS have abdominal pain, but the key to its cause lies in the nature of the stools, as we shall see in the next chapter.

SUMMARY

➤ Think hard about your symptoms, so that you can give your doctor an accurate description.

➤ Where do you feel abdominal pain?

➤ When do you feel abdominal pain, and what makes it worse – or better?

➤ How often do you need to go to the lavatory?

➤ Do you have to rush to go, for fear of having 'an accident'?

➤ Or do you strain to pass anything at all?

➤ Look closely at the stools you pass and compare them with the Bristol Stool Form Scale (page 26).

CHAPTER 3

Which Sort of IBS Do You Have?

You might be forgiven for thinking that IBS is quite unlike other medical conditions – that it is some sort of bizarre and incomprehensible process far beyond the wit of man, which will never be understood or successfully treated. This is quite wrong. IBS is just like any other disorder, and managed according to the same principles. It is necessary to find the cause of the problem, and then deal with it in a logical way.

This is not always easy, because the causes of IBS vary immensely. Large drug companies spend millions of pounds on developing 'a treatment for IBS', but no drug has ever been discovered that is effective in every case and nor will one ever be. Sadly, most of the products presently available are of little use in any case. If this were not true you would not now be bothering to read this book. Because of this self-evident fact, we shan't waste any space discussing the pharmaceutical products for IBS that are currently on the market.

Furthermore, many doctors do not yet differentiate between one form of IBS and another. This again is a recipe for failure, because if you don't know a precise cause you can never recommend a precise treatment. Back in the 1980s we found that many of our IBS patients were dramatically better when we changed their diets, switching to low fibre or excluding certain foods. We thought that we had the answer to IBS. Foolish dreams! We soon discovered that some patients did not benefit at all from what we recommended. Clearly, the cases that responded to diet were merely a proportion (albeit a large proportion – up to 65 per cent) of a much bigger group. However, when we were able to take away the cases that responded successfully to diet, those remaining, which did not get better on diet, could be separated much more clearly. Slowly, the pieces of the jigsaw started to fall into place.

Some cases of IBS were associated with marked anxiety. Anxiety itself can give rise to many symptoms (as will be discussed in Chapter 7), but it frequently causes patients to breathe more rapidly and to swallow air. The air then expands the stomach and passes down the gut, leading to pain, rumbling, bloating and wind. Treating these cases with diet did no good at all as it tended to make patients even more anxious, particularly when they found they were not getting any better.

We also discovered that, in some patients, abdominal pain arose not from the bowel at all, but from pressure on the nerves leaving the spine that supply the abdominal wall, or from damage to the muscles in the abdominal wall. This problem is discussed in detail in Chapter 11. With female patients, some of their bowel symptoms arise at differing stages of the menstrual cycle, often just before the period is due or in mid-cycle, after ovulation. The link between the menstrual cycle and the gut is discussed in Chapter 10.

We noticed that most patients who got better on our diets suffered from diarrhoea. This was often urgent and usually frequent, occurring several times a week. But there were some patients with diarrhoea for whom the diet was of dubious value. After starting their diets, they might not have diarrhoea for several days, but then suddenly their attacks returned. The links between the symptoms and the foods they were eating were uncertain.

Some patients struggled with diets for weeks and months, trying to sort out their IBS, but with little success.

THE DIETARY APPROACH

One recent change in the classification of IBS has been to divide patients according to whether abdominal pain was accompanied by diarrhoea (called IBS-D), constipation (IBS-C), or by alternation between the two (IBS-A). But we found these changes were of little or no help in deciding which of our patients would be most suitable for dietary treatment. Some logical way to sort out IBS patients was essential. Gillian Kirby, one of our dietitians at Addenbrooke's Hospital, devised a schedule (shown below) based on the broad principles that:

➤ Patients with diarrhoea and wind needed dietary help.

➤ Patients with constipation needed fibre.

➤ Patients with constipation associated with excess wind needed a low-fibre diet and bulk laxatives.

➤ Patients with diarrhoea and alternating constipation/diarrhoea were treated first with changes in fibre, and if this was ineffective with an exclusion diet, to avoid foods that seemed to trigger symptoms.

DIETARY SCHEDULE FOR IBS AS USED AT ADDENBROOKE'S HOSPITAL

SYMPTOMS	DIET
Constipation without bloating or wind	High fibre
Constipation with bloating and wind	Low fibre with bulking agent
Diarrhoea without bloating or wind	First: Low fibre – if diet already high in fibre Second: Exclusion – if diet already low in fibre
Diarrhoea with bloating and wind	First: Low fibre Second: Exclusion
Alternating constipation/diarrhoea without bloating or wind	First: High fibre or bulking agent Second: Exclusion
Alternating constipation/diarrhoea with bloating and wind	First: Low fibre with bulking agent Second: Exclusion

This system worked so well we were able to set up a clinic at Addenbrooke's for IBS patients under the age of 40, run by dietitians alone. By reading the referral letters from GPs, consultants initially decided which patients were suitable to attend the dietitian-led clinic. To exclude other diseases of the gut the patients were then asked to provide blood and stool samples and to complete a questionnaire seeking symptoms of anxiety. They were then asked to come to the clinic a few days later, when the results of these tests would be available to the dietitian.

If all results were normal, the dietitians treated the patients according to the scheme set out above. If the tests showed any abnormalities, the dietitians would send the patient to one of the doctors in the clinic to take over and investigate in detail. Otherwise, none of the medical staff was involved in any way.

The dietitian-led clinic proved very successful. No one complained that he or she was being seen by a dietitian rather than a doctor, and in the first year over 61 per cent of patients seen at the clinic found that their symptoms were reduced by at least half. A couple of years later the success rate had risen to 70 per cent. The clinic now runs every week at Addenbrooke's, saving a great deal of time and expense. It has led to a marked shortening in waiting lists for appointments in the gastroenterology out-patients department.

A CHANGE OF APPROACH

In 1999, however, new research changed our approach to IBS patients dramatically. Two doctors working in Sweden, Doctors Ragnarsson and Bodemar, studied 108 patients with IBS in great detail. The patients compiled symptom-diaries for six weeks, recording pain, wind, diarrhoea, bloating and stool habit. Symptoms were then analysed using a sophisticated computer programme. This showed that IBS patients could be separated into three quite different groups, based on bowel habit, rather than differences in pain, bloating and wind (which they all suffered).

➤ **Group 1**: painful intermittent diarrhoea – every 7–14 days. In between attacks, stools were small, hard and pellet-like and the patient often needed to strain to pass them.

➤ **Group 2**: loose, urgent stools most of the time and attacks of diarrhoea on three or more days each week.

➤ **Group 3**: bowel habits were virtually normal.

Group 1 corresponded closely to the group for whom changes in diet had not helped. The small and hard stools that Group 1 patients passed between each bout of diarrhoea suggested that they were basically constipated. Over a few days, the amount of faecal matter lying in the bowel increased and when it reached a certain threshold, an attack of diarrhoea could be triggered.

All sorts of different events might trigger an attack, including stress, rich or heavy meals, exercise, travel or tiredness. The bowel would be left virtually empty by the bout of diarrhoea and then several days would elapse as the bowel filled up again, before a further attack of diarrhoea could follow. We decided to put this theory to the test.

We devised a questionnaire based on Ragnarsson and Bodemar's classification and selected patients for treatment according to their scores. If they scored highly for Group 1, they would be given laxatives to overcome the underlying constipation. If they scored highly for Group 2, they would be given a low fibre or exclusion diet. Patients who fell into Group 3 (with pain, bloating and wind but normal bowel habits) completed two further questionnaires, one to check for anxiety and air swallowing and one to check for musculo-skeletal pain (that is, pain affecting the bones or muscles). All 61 IBS patients recruited for our study fell into one or other of Ragnarsson and Bodemar's three groups. The results were:

➤ **Group 1**: 15 patients –12 were relieved by laxatives.

➤ **Group 2**: 28 patients – 21 were relieved by diet.

➤ **Group 3**: 18 patients – 12 patients had anxiety and air-swallowing: seven reported improvement; six patients had musculo-skeletal pain; four recovered.

These success rates were considerably higher than those that we have reported in previous studies of the treatment of IBS. Nevertheless, 20–25 per cent of patients still responded poorly, perhaps due to other causes of IBS as yet undiscovered or because they didn't follow the treatment. In the treatment of IBS, what you get out depends on what you put in. There is no golden bullet to make matters simple, and if you wish to be control your IBS you have to work at it consistently.

However, our questionnaires provided a reliable way of dividing the patients into groups for which logical treatment is available and showed that it is possible to control IBS symptoms in the great majority of IBS patients. The aim of this book is to make this knowledge available to a wider group of IBS sufferers.

GETTING STARTED

The crucial question in managing your IBS is to decide what is your predominant stool habit. You will need to record your stool pattern carefully for perhaps seven to 10 days, or even more if you are badly constipated. Recording your stool habit will determine whether you need to progress to our questionnaire for determining the possible causes of your IBS, or whether you need to turn to Chapter 8 on Constipation. Women should try to avoid recording their stool pattern during the week coming up to their period, as this may be unrepresentative.

Examine each stool, and classify it according to the Bristol Stool Form Scale (page 26). Write the score down, until you have accumulated at least a dozen separate stool results. You should then see which stool form predominates. If at least 50 per cent of your stools fall into the same category it will give a reasonable guide to your whole gut transit time (WGTT), and help you choose the next step of your treatment. If less than 50 per cent are the same, use the predominant type – as long as it is greater than 25 per cent it will be reasonably accurate.

If you have had a definite attack of loose, urgent diarrhoea during your stool recording period, do not worry about the Bristol score. Instead, go to the questionnaire on page 38 and determine your scores for fermentation, and for overload and overflow.

If you have **not** had a definite attack of loose diarrhoea, then go by the Bristol Stool Form Scale. If your predominant score is 1 or 2 on the Bristol Scale you are constipated, so go directly to Chapter 8 on Constipation. If your predominant Bristol Scale score is 3 or higher, complete the questionnaire.

When you have completed the questionnaire you will have a score for each of the following categories of IBS – fermentation, overload and overflow, air-swallowing and musculo-skeletal pain. Positive scores are:

Fermentation	11 or more (see Chapter 5)
Overload and overflow	11 or more (see Chapter 6)
Musculo-skeletal	5 or more (see Chapter 11)
Air-swallowing	24 or more (see Chapter 7)
Menstrual problems	6 or more (see Chapter 10)

If you are positive for a single category, go to the chapter dealing with it, and follow the guidance provided. If you are positive for more than one category, read Chapter 4 before deciding which aspect of your IBS to attack first.

If you are a woman of child-bearing age, you should also complete the menstrual section. Probably the questionnaire has already revealed that you are positive for another type of IBS. If so, you should approach this first, and you may find that you get a welcome surprise about its effects on your cycle. If not, or if symptoms persist after following the treatment advised, read Chapter 10 for further suggestions.

IBS QUESTIONNAIRES

You now need to complete the following questionnaires and add up your scores for each section. Decide which description of the frequency of your symptoms fits best. Base your symptoms on their frequency in the previous month. Don't classify any symptoms as falling between two categories, as this will invalidate the scoring. Don't use any medication for your IBS while monitoring your symptoms as this may distort the picture. You may find that the diary of your bowel habits that you prepared to calculate the Bristol Stool Form Scale (page 26) helps with questions 1 and 3.

Remember that if your predominant Bristol score was only 1 or 2 – that is to say you suffer predominant constipation – *go straight to Chapter 8 on Constipation*. If however, you suffer diarrhoea (even infrequently) complete the questionnaires below.

When completing the questionnaires, the scores are defined as follows:

Never	you never have this symptom
Rare	you have this symptom once every 2–3 months
Sometimes	you have this symptom 2–3 times a month
Often	you have this symptom once or twice a week
Very often	you have this symptom 3–4 times a week or more

Note: this is not applicable to question 13.

1. **Are your stools loose and runny?**

Never	Rarely	Sometimes	Often	Very often
0	0	1	1	2

2. **Are your stools hard and pellet like?**

Never	Rarely	Sometimes	Often	Very often
4	3	2	1	0

3. **Do you have to rush to the lavatory to open your bowels with great urgency?**

Never	Rarely	Sometimes	Often	Very often
0	1	2	3	4

4. **Do you ever have to strain or push to pass a motion?**

Never	Rarely	Sometimes	Often	Very often
4	3	2	1	0

5. **Do you ever feel that you have not emptied your bowels completely?**

Never	Rarely	Sometimes	Often	Very often
4	3	2	1	0

If you score 11 or more on questions 1–5 you suffer from malfermentation: see page 53.

6. **Are your stools loose and runny?**

Never	Rarely	Sometimes	Often	Very often
0	1	2	3	4

7. **Are your stools sometimes hard and pellet-like?**

Never	Rarely	Sometimes	Often	Very often
0	1	2	3	4

8. **Do you have to rush to the lavatory to open your bowels with great urgency?**

Never	Rarely	Sometimes	Often	Very often
0	3	3	0	0

9. Do you ever have to strain or push to pass a motion?

Never	Rarely	Sometimes	Often	Very often
0	1	2	3	4

10. Do you ever feel that you have not emptied your bowels completely?

Never	Rarely	Sometimes	Often	Very often
0	1	2	3	4

If you score 11 or more on questions 6–10 you suffer from overload and overflow: see page 87.

11. Does coughing, sneezing or taking a deep breath make the pain worse?

Never	Rarely	Sometimes	Often	Very often
0	1	2	3	4

12. Does bending, sitting, lifting, twisting or turning over in bed make the pain worse?

Never	Rarely	Sometimes	Often	Very often
0	1	2	3	4

If you score 5 or more on questions 11 and 12 you suffer from musculo-skeletal pain: see page 165.

The following section is for women of childbearing age who are NOT pregnant:

If you have had a hysterectomy answer questions 8–10.

If you are still menstruating answer questions 11–13.

DO NOT ANSWER BOTH SETS OF QUESTIONS.

If you have had a hysterectomy:

13. Was either ovary left in place?

Yes	No
2	0

14. Do you suffer from breast soreness?

Never	Rarely	Sometimes	Often	Very often
0	1	2	3	4

15. If you have pain or diarrhoea, does it come just before or during the time when your breasts are tender?

Never	Rarely	Sometimes	Often	Very often
0	1	2	3	4

If you are still menstruating:

16. If you have IBS pain, is it related to your menstrual cycle?

Never	Rarely	Sometimes	Often	Very often
0	1	2	3	4

17. Do you notice any change in your bowel habit just before or during your period?

Never	Rarely	Sometimes	Often	Very often
0	1	2	3	4

18. Do you suffer from PMT?

Never	Rarely	Sometimes	Often	Very often
0	1	2	3	4

If you score 6 or more on questions 13–15 or 16 –18 you suffer from menstrual problems: see page 159.

The following questionnaire is simpler. Just tick the frequency of each symptom and add up your total using the number given:

	Never	Rarely	Sometimes	Often	Very often
Chest pain	0	1	2	3	4
Feeling tense	0	1	2	3	4
Blurred vision	0	1	2	3	4
Dizzy spells	0	1	2	3	4
Feeling confused	0	1	2	3	4
Faster or deeper breathing	0	1	2	3	4
Short of breath	0	1	2	3	4
Tight feelings in the chest	0	1	2	3	4
Bloated feelings in the stomach	0	1	2	3	4
Tingling fingers	0	1	2	3	4
Unable to breathe deeply	0	1	2	3	4
Stiff fingers or arms	0	1	2	3	4

	Never	Rarely	Sometimes	Often	Very Often
Tight feelings around mouth	0	1	2	3	4
Cold hands or feet	0	1	2	3	4
Heart racing (palpitation)	0	1	2	3	4
Feelings of anxiety	0	1	2	3	4

Based on Nijmegen Questionnaire (van Dixhoorn and Duivenvoorden, 1985)

If you score 24 or more you suffer from anxiety and air swallowing: see page 97.

If you are positive for a single form of IBS, turn to the relevant chapter to discover how to control it. If you are positive for two or more forms, you should first read Chapter 4 to decide which part of the problem to control first.

KEEP A FOOD AND LIFESTYLE DIARY

It may be helpful to keep a diary recording when and what you eat and drink, together with a record of your symptoms. Include details such as periods of increased anxiety and the phase of your menstrual cycle. Anxiety can over-stimulate the gut and lead to air swallowing causing bloating and distension. This matter is dealt with in detail in Chapter 7. Changes in the hormone levels during the menstrual cycle may play an important role, too. This is further discussed in Chapter 10. This should help you determine whether there are any links between these factors and your symptoms.

CHANGING YOUR LIFESTYLE

Depending on the form of IBS you have found yourself to be suffering from, it may be necessary to treat your symptoms by following a special diet. Before embarking on such a diet, however, it is worth considering simple, more general changes to your diet and lifestyle that may have important benefits. For example, if you tend to skip meals and grab a snack when time permits, or if you eat very quickly or don't drink enough clear fluid or drink coffee and tea continually throughout the day, your gut may not be able to function as efficiently as it should.

➤ **Develop a regular meal pattern.** This will help your gut establish its own routine. If meals are missed, signals that regulate bowel movements become confused. A large meal on a stomach that has been starved most of the day may result in an exaggerated stimulus to the bowels and can in turn lead to discomfort and diarrhoea.

➤ **Eat little and often.** Spread your food intake evenly throughout the day. If during a meal your stomach starts to feel uncomfortable, stop eating – save the pudding until later. Some people find four or five small meals and snacks easier to manage than two or three large ones.

➤ **Take time when you eat.** Eating quickly and drinking fluids at the same time makes it more likely that you will swallow air, leading to bloating and flatulence. Rushing around after eating diverts the blood away from gut to the muscles and this too may disrupt digestion.

➤ **Have regular drinks.** Aim for a minimum of eight cups or glasses a day. This is particularly important if you have constipation. Fibrous matter in the intestine absorbs water, making it swell. This produces a bulky stool that helps stimulate the bowel muscles to push its contents through the system. If you are dehydrated, stools will be small and hard, making them difficult to pass. Try to include drinks such as water, fruit juice and squashes. Some people find that carbonated drinks cause bloating and discomfort.

➤ **Avoid caffeine.** This is found in coffee, tea and cola drinks and can act as a powerful stimulus to the gut and make it difficult to relax intestinal muscles. Try to reduce caffeine intake by replacing with decaffeinated varieties or herbal and fruit teas.

➤ **Avoid stomach irritants.** Very spicy foods, acidic foods (citrus foods or vinegar), and some raw vegetables such as cucumbers, peppers and onions can irritate the stomach. Alcohol too can act as an irritant, particularly on an empty stomach. Fried and very rich foods are common causes of indigestion and heartburn. It's also important to consider the amount of fibre you are eating – too much or too little. We will discuss this in more detail later on.

SUMMARY

➤ Not all IBS-like symptoms are due to IBS – sometimes the problem involves damage to bones and/or muscles, or is related to anxiety and air swallowing.

➤ In women, IBS-like symptoms may be due to – or made worse by – menstrual problems.

➤ Increasing or decreasing fibre can help many IBS sufferers – but not all.

➤ Some IBS sufferers benefit from excluding problem foods.

➤ Before you make radical changes to your diet, see whether simple lifestyle changes can help.

➤ Answer the questionnaire to identify which form(s) of IBS you are suffering from, or whether other factors play a part, and then turn to the relevant chapter(s).

CHAPTER 4

What If You Have Two or More Forms of IBS?

Whenever a remedy for IBS has been suggested, there have been patients who did not respond to it. The whole purpose of this book has been to try to create order out of this confusion and suggest how a logical analysis of symptoms can lead to the application of a suitable, successful treatment regime.

Nevertheless, although I have divided IBS according to its various causes, such as anxiety, malfermentation or constipation, there are difficult cases that do not fit snugly into one particular pattern. This is usually not because they are due to some entirely separate cause, but because more than one form of IBS is present in the same person.

CASE STUDY

A woman of 35 was referred to me following extensive gynaecological surgery including the removal of the uterus and one of her ovaries. She had developed severe abdominal pain and diarrhoea. Initially, this was treated by excluding wheat and milk from her diet with considerable success and her diarrhoea settled. However, after only a few weeks of improved health, she developed further symptoms of pain, wind and bloating and on her next visit it became clear that she had developed anxiety and over-breathing (hyperventilation) with considerable

---

air swallowing. She was treated successfully as described in Chapter 7 and for some months she remained without symptoms.

Then her abdominal pain returned, this time with constipation. Linseed was added to her diet and the constipation was cured. A few months later she was in trouble again with intermittent bouts of abdominal pain and diarrhoea. As she had had a hysterectomy, she no longer had menstrual periods, but her attacks were cyclical and coincided with breast soreness. As she still retained one functioning ovary, her monthly hormone pattern was continuing, and it therefore seemed likely her IBS was related to menstruation. A medication (Zoladex) was implanted under her skin to inhibit her ovarian hormones and this rapidly cured her symptoms.

She now continues well on her wheat- and milk-free diet supplemented by daily doses of linseed. After the effects of the first implant wore off, her ovarian hormones were kept under control by an intra-uterine contraceptive device (IUCD or coil) releasing local progesterone, together with an oestrogen patch.

Thus to control this woman's IBS completely, it was necessary to use several different forms of treatment. At the time that I saw this patient, we were not using questionnaires – we just picked things up as we went along. We now know that some of our patients score positive results in more than one part of the questionnaire. The commonest is for anxiety with malfermentation or overload and overflow. So which type of IBS should be treated first?

The basic principle underlying the approach to treatment is to try simple things first, and more complex matters later. Thus, it's obviously much easier to take a bulk laxative to ease constipation than it is to follow an exclusion diet. Anxiety, however, is so important in IBS that it over-rides most other considerations. This is not because it is the commonest cause of IBS, or produces the worst symptoms – it isn't and it doesn't.

Many patients with IBS that originally arose from different causes also become anxious later because their problem is not skilfully and sympathetically handled by the doctors they first meet. A study in the USA suggested that anxiety was quite uncommon in patients who were seen for the first time shortly after the onset of IBS. But in patients coming to the clinic after IBS had been present for five years or more anxiety frequently developed because their symptoms had persisted with no effective treatment.

Furthermore, symptoms produced by anxiety are very easily triggered in susceptible people. Relatively slight deviations from the normal routine at work, in their social lives or even in their diets may be sufficient to make anxious patients breathe more rapidly, swallow air and develop symptoms. This can often be seen when patients with anxiety try to follow an exclusion diet.

Effects caused by anxiety can easily be mistakenly attributed to a specific food that is being tested – and they frequently are! This is the usual reason that some patients believe that they are upset by a vast range of foods and chemicals. Their IBS is caused by something completely different, such as anxiety, but they blame the food they are eating every time they begin to feel unwell. It then becomes difficult, if not impossible, to find a diet that is nutritionally adequate. I therefore believe anxiety must be tackled first.

As explained in Chapter 7, one of the main reasons that anxiety leads to IBS is because it promotes air swallowing. The key to its successful management is to reduce air swallowing by re-training breathing habits and ensuring that the nasal airway is clear.

Unfortunately, this takes time, practice and perseverance in order to bring it completely under control. However, such an approach enables you to understand how dramatically changes in breathing can produce gut symptoms. When this is appreciated, it becomes much easier to put matters in perspective and not to keep blaming the onset of belly-aches on some exotic constituent in the previous meal.

If anxiety is associated with marked diarrhoea, it is often sensible to go on a low-fibre gluten-free diet (page 78) at the same time as you are starting breathing exercises for anxiety. If the diarrhoea improves, the anxiety state will lessen and will be controlled more easily. However, it is always a mistake to try reintroducing foods while anxiety persists. It is then very easy to blame foods for symptoms caused by anxiety, so keep to the basic diet until you have got your breathing under control.

When anxiety is not present or when it has been satisfactorily dealt with, other problems should be approached by trying the simplest treatments first. Treat problems associated with constipation (Chapter 8) before those related to malfermentation (Chapter 5), as that will require, at least at first, a limited diet with the social difficulties that this may cause. In the case of musculo-skeletal and menstrual problems, however, malfermentation should be corrected first. Many women find that menstrually related symptoms improve with diet. This is also true of a small number of musculo-skeletal syndromes.

Clearly, if you only score positive in one part of the questionnaire, get on straight away with the treatment recommended. If you score positive in two or more, however, treat them in the order with which they come in the list below:

1.   Overload and overflow – bulk laxatives are easy (see page 87).
2.   Anxiety and air swallowing – get your breathing under control to avoid confusion (see pages 97, 99).
3.   Constipation – page 119.
4.   Malfermentation – page 53.
5.   Musculo-skeletal problems – page 165.
6.   Menstrual difficulties (when relevant) – page 159.

WHAT IF I SEEM TO BE POSITIVE FOR NEARLY EVERYTHING?

In my experience it is extremely unusual for patients to score positive for three or more causes. However, if you feel overwhelmed and totally confused and don't know where to turn, then this bit is for you!

In the first instance, try a low-fibre gluten-free diet, supplemented by a bulk laxative such as Normacol or linseed (after a bowel clear out – see page 89) to relieve any constipation, while at the same time undertaking breathing retraining (see page 99). You will inevitably start to feel better quite quickly and, as symptoms clear, you will be able to use the knowledge of IBS that you have gleaned from this book to appreciate the reasons for those that persist.

If you seem to get stuck, try doing the questionnaire again – using your latest set of symptoms. This often shows the best way to get back on track. If you come to realise that you are still having problems with anxiety, you may need to enlist the help of a specialist physiotherapist, or if the problem is malfermentation, to try a formal exclusion diet.

The key is to keep thinking about the symptoms you suffer and to keep on trying to explain them on the basis of your knowledge of IBS. Remember, knowledge is power!

SUMMARY

➤ IBS symptoms can have more than one cause, either at the same time or one after the other.

➤ If your questionnaire scores suggest this applies to you, tackle anxiety first as this can override all other causes – see page 97.

➤ Then tackle your problems in turn, using the easiest measures first.

➤ Use bulk laxatives if you suffer from overload and overflow – see page 91.

➤ Control your breathing to reduce air swallowing – see page 99.

➤ Manage constipation (page 119) before malfermentation – see page 53.

➤ Finally, tackle musculo-skeletal and menstrual problems – see page 165 and page 159.

CHAPTER 5

Malfermentation and IBS

If, after completing the questionnaire, you find you have a high score for malfermentation, here is the place to begin! The likeliest cause of your symptoms is food intolerance. One of the most common intolerances in IBS patients is to fibre. We will look at other causes later on.

FIBRE AND MALFERMENTATION

The UK diet tends to contain a lot of highly processed and convenience foods that are very low in fibre. Fibre is found in whole-grain breads, cereals, vegetables, pulses (beans, lentils and peas), fruits, nuts and seeds. These foods are important not only because they contribute vitamins and minerals to the diet but also because fibre itself has an important role. It absorbs fluid from the gut, which makes it swell, producing a soft stool that is easy to pass. The increased stool bulk helps to stimulate the bowel wall to contract and so pushes the contents through. Fibre has other benefits, too. It reduces the absorption of cholesterol (so protecting against heart disease), reduces the risk of gallstones and helps prevent diverticular disease and piles.

In the 1970s, doctors throughout the country recommended high-fibre diets enthusiastically for patients with IBS – especially extra bran. However, at Addenbrooke's, many of our patients said that bran made their symptoms worse. They were suffering from more wind and bloating and in many cases diarrhoea had become more frequent. So, while there is little doubt that a high-fibre diet may prove very helpful where IBS is associated with constipation (see Chapter 8), we no longer believe that this is true for the majority of IBS sufferers.

Foods that tend to make wind and bloating worse include dried fruits and nuts such as almonds, certain beans including baked beans, and other vegetables including brassicas – broccoli, cabbage, cauliflower and Brussels sprouts. Beer and other fizzy drinks such as lemonade and cola drinks can also increase wind and bloating. Wheat fibre is particularly difficult and may be found in bran, wholemeal and whole-grain bread products, muesli and pastry (where fat is also a problem). Pulses (peas and beans) contain certain sugars that cannot be digested and are renowned for producing excessive wind!

We came up with a very simple idea. If high-fibre diets seemed to make IBS worse, why don't we try low-fibre diets instead? Happily, when we tried this approach many of our patients reported considerable improvement. We even received a letter from a female patient who told us that a low-fibre diet had settled the diarrhoea from which she had suffered for over 20 years, despite the best efforts of several distinguished physicians. But this didn't explain why fibre was causing problems.

BACTERIAL FERMENTATION

A drug called Enterovioform, used to treat bacterial gastroenteritis, was found to help many patients with food intolerance. Unfortunately it had serious side effects and has now been withdrawn, but it showed that reducing bacterial activity in the bowel could help patients with this problem. It was also discovered that patients often felt very much better having had a bowel clearout in preparation for a barium enema or colonoscopy. Furthermore, some patients with severe food intolerance found they were temporarily much improved after a course of antibiotics, prescribed for an incidental infection. This suggested that we should concentrate on the bacteria in the gut as a likely cause of this problem.

There is now an impressive body of evidence suggesting that the type of IBS associated with food intolerance is caused by abnormal fermentation by gut bacteria, which we call malfermentation. Studies carried out in Italy (and confirmed by us) have shown that, although there are no specific disease-causing (pathogenic) bacteria in the stools of these patients, the bacteria in their bowel are different from those of normal individuals. The numbers of *Lactobacilli* and *Bifidobacter* and *Escherichia coli* are reduced.

We also found an increase in the numbers of a group of bacteria normally only present in small numbers in the gut because they prefer to live in the presence of oxygen – of which there is very little in the bowel. Although these bacteria (called facultative anaerobes) prefer to grow in oxygen they can exist without it. Not only were their numbers much greater in patients with IBS than in non-sufferers, but they increased as much as 100-fold following a diet that included sufficient wheat to provoke symptoms.

These studies strongly supported our suspicion that bacteria were important in food intolerance. We examined the stools of many patients over a series of months and found the bacterial population in IBS patients to be very unstable. In normal individuals, once a healthy bacterial flora is established in infancy, it tends to remain constant with very few changes until the patient reaches old age.

By contrast, in IBS it changes from week to week and even from day to day, with bacteria coming and going in apparently random fashion. It seemed likely to us that this was the result of the loss of important species of bacteria from the healthy flora, thus allowing other bacteria that happened to be passing through the bowel to move in. As these bacteria were not truly part of the normal flora for that individual, they were eliminated after a few days, only for another passing species to take their place.

This problem has also been examined in a different way. A study at St George's Hospital in London involved patients who did not suffer from IBS, but who were given antibiotics to treat infection. They were followed up a year later and compared with those who had not received antibiotic treatment during the preceding year. The risk of developing IBS in the following year was four times greater in the antibiotic-treated group than in the others. This showed that treatment with antibiotics can damage the gut flora and lead to IBS.

Far more likely to provoke IBS, however, is gastrointestinal infection. The Infectious Diseases Department in Sheffield followed up patients who had suffered gastroenteritis and found that many went on to develop IBS. A larger study, performed in Spain, showed that patients who had gastroenteritis were nearly 12 times more likely to develop IBS in the subsequent year than others. IBS may also follow other treatments such as anaesthetics or radiotherapy that can damage bowel bacteria.

We had already shown that Crohn's disease could be controlled by diet in a similar way to IBS. We needed to do further tests to see if any differences could be shown between bacterial activity in IBS and in healthy people. We decided to measure hydrogen and methane production in IBS patients and non-sufferers – both gases are produced by gut bacteria. All gases released from the breath and rectum were collected by having subjects lie in a bed surrounded by a plastic cover over an aluminium frame.

For two weeks the two groups were given a standard British diet. At the end of this time the subjects went into the tent and their gas excretion was measured over 24 hours. Then they were given two weeks off to eat whatever they chose before starting on an exclusion diet in which wheat, cereal fibre and milk were replaced by fruit and vegetables including soya. Again, after two weeks, the volunteers were studied over a second 24-hour period. It was found that when the IBS patients were put on the exclusion diet, the production of hydrogen dropped to around one-eighth of its original level and their symptoms improved. Thus by changing the diet it was possible to change the activity of the gut bacteria.

At the end of both 24-hour study periods, the patients were asked to drink some lactulose. This is a sugar that can't be digested and so passes into the large intestine where it is fermented by bacteria, releasing hydrogen and methane. These gases were then measured on breath samples over three hours. The amount of hydrogen excreted on the breath in both groups was greater when they were following the standard diet than when they were on the exclusion diet. At the same time methane excretion in the breath tended to increase on the exclusion diet. This was strong evidence that the diet was influencing bacterial activity. Other studies provided further proof of the crucial importance of these bacteria in food intolerance.

FIBRE – HOW MUCH DO WE NEED?

This seemed to pose something of a problem. Fibre is needed for good gut health, and yet in some IBS sufferers, fibre such as bran is fermented in the large bowel, resulting in excessive gas, bloating, flatulence and discomfort. Too much fibre may also aggravate diarrhoea. Ideally we should all take 25–30 g daily, but, in the presence of malfermentation, an increase in fibre intake usually makes matters worse.

Fortunately, we can get around this problem by using bulking agents. These are natural sources of fibre that cannot be broken down to any extent by bacteria in the gut. Thus they have the beneficial effects of fibre without making gas and diarrhoea worse. The benefits of a high-fibre diet for those IBS patients with constipation are discussed in detail in Chapter 8, and other points regarding the use of fibre are discussed on pages 62–63. But fibre is a problem in only some IBS patients who are intolerant to foods. What are the other foods that might be triggering symptoms – and why?

EXCLUDING PROBLEM FOODS

To look for specific foods upsetting the bowel in IBS we switched from using the low-fibre diet to an elimination diet. Here the patient starts off by eating a single meat such as lamb or turkey and a single fruit such as pear or melon together with an easily digestible source of carbohydrate such as rice, all washed down with water.

During the first two to three days of the diet, the patient frequently felt very unwell with headaches, general aching, abdominal pains and sometimes even vomiting. However, these symptoms passed by the third or fourth day and patients then began to feel steadily better. When all the symptoms had cleared, perhaps after seven to 10 days, foods were re-introduced slowly one at a time to see which, if any, triggered IBS symptoms. We then carried out further studies that confirmed the success of this approach.

For some months we treated all patients with IBS with this rigorous elimination diet, which became known as the 'Lamb and Pears' regime. Of 172 patients treated, no less than 122 gained complete control of their symptoms, and nor was this just a short-term benefit. When we sent follow-up postal questionnaires to the patients three years after we had treated them, we found that over 90 per cent were still following their diets and remained in perfect control of their IBS.

Nevertheless, the elimination diet was a major problem for patients. The necessity to keep to lamb, pears and rice for several days was a real difficulty. Some patients' withdrawal symptoms when the diet was started were so bad that we had to take them into hospital and give them intravenous fluids to get through the period of pain and vomiting. With increasing experience, we were starting to get to know the foods most likely to upset our patients. From this list we developed a less restrictive exclusion diet that avoided all the foods that had upset at least 20 per cent or more of our patients.

This list was modified slightly following two subsequent reviews of the diet to produce the exclusion diet that we recommend to this day. Altogether 584 patients with IBS took part in these studies and approximately 60 per cent found that they were able to control these symptoms on this diet.

PROBLEM FOODS MOST LIKELY TO UPSET OUR PATIENTS

FOODS	% AFFECTED	FOODS	% AFFECTED
Cereals		**Vegetables**	
Wheat	60	Onions	22
Corn	44	Potatoes	20
Oats	34		
Rye	30	**Fruit**	
Barley	24	Citrus	24
Dairy Products		**Miscellaneous**	
Milk	44	Coffee	33
Cheese	39	Tea	25
Eggs	26	Nuts	22
Butter	25	Chocolate	22
Yoghurt	24	Preservatives	20
		Yeast	20

WHY DO FOODS UPSET THE GUT?

We now knew from our studies that in many people IBS symptoms were genuine responses to food. This had been confirmed by the release of chemicals in the rectum called prostaglandins that may trigger symptoms such as pain and diarrhoea. We also knew that many of our patients had remained well for up to three years by excluding problem foods. The question now was why?

We carried out further studies, often involving experts in relevant fields, to discover whether food allergy or intolerance to lactose, the sugar found in milk, may be factors in IBS. First, allergy tests were performed to determine whether IBS patients had genuine allergies to the foods that upset them, but these proved negative. Next we turned our attention to lactose intolerance. This is caused by a deficiency of lactase – the enzyme needed to digest milk sugar (lactose). It is very common in adults of non-Caucasian origin but Europeans can sometimes suffer this problem too.

In a study of 127 patients with IBS (mostly Northern Europeans), we were surprised to find that the number who had low levels of lactase was quite high – about 25 per cent. This is in keeping with similar studies from other centres. However, lactase deficiency in itself was not sufficient to account for these patients developing IBS.

We put the patients lacking the enzyme on low lactose diets and found that only about one third of them improved. When we put them on exclusion diets, however, over half of them responded and some found that they were upset by cow's milk. As these patients had not felt better after following the low lactose diet, it followed that another component of cow's milk, apart from lactose – such as milk fat – must be the culprit. But this was still only a minority of patients.

WHICH DIET SHOULD I CHOOSE?

There are basically two forms of diet that will reduce malfermentation. As we have shown, one is the low-fibre diet and the other is the exclusion diet. Some experts recommend a low-fibre diet that is also free of gluten (the protein found in wheat and other cereal products), so all three diets are included here.

LOW-FIBRE DIET

This is probably the most straightforward of those we use in the treatment of IBS. For this reason, it is usually the first tried in the Dietitian-led Clinic at Addenbrooke's and it proves very successful. If your questionnaire scores have suggested you suffer from malfermentation, you should try the low-fibre diet first – unless, when you look through the diet sheet (page 63), you see that you are already following a diet that is low in fibre. Of course, if you can see a dietitian, he or she will be able to give you definite advice on this point. If you are already on a low-fibre diet, then try the exclusion diet (page 66) instead.

Follow the low-fibre diet for four weeks. If you don't notice an improvement in your symptoms or you feel worse at this time, then return to your usual diet. If, however, you are feeling better, try to reintroduce some fibre into your diet, following the guidelines on page 64.

Sometimes patients find that they tolerate some types of fibre better than others and it's therefore necessary to reintroduce these separately to note their effects. Build up the fibre to a level that you can tolerate. If you are unable to reintroduce much fibre, you may need a vitamin and mineral supplement to ensure your diet is balanced. This should be discussed with a dietitian.

If you find that the low-fibre diet tends to make you constipated, take a bulking agent (bulk laxative). It would be sensible to discuss this with your GP. Bulking agents are natural sources of fibre that cannot be broken down by bacteria in the gut. This means that they encourage regular bowel movement but – in contrast to cereal, vegetable and fruit fibre – do not contribute to gas production.

There are several suitable varieties. Those that are least likely to be broken down by bacteria include linseed (available from health food shops), Normacol (sterculia) and methyl cellulose. Initially linseed and sterculia are probably the best bulking agents to try as methyl cellulose sometimes slows up gut transit and makes constipation worse. However, if your stools still tend to be a little loose and frequent, then methyl cellulose could be the agent to choose.

We no longer recommend laxatives based on ispaghula husk (Fybogel, Regulan, Psyllium, Isogel) as this can be broken down by gut bacteria and can sometimes cause excess gas and bloating. If one variety does not suit you, it's worth trying an alternative.

It's essential that you drink extra fluids when taking bulk laxatives to enable them to work properly.

LOW-FIBRE DIET SHEET

Eat your usual amount of meat, fish, eggs, milk and dairy products and fats and oils. These do not contain any fibre. For cereal products, fruits and vegetables follow the guidelines below:

PRODUCT	NOT ALLOWED	ALLOWED
Cereal	Wholemeal, granary and brown bread, bran, wholemeal flour and foods made with these	White bread, white flour and foods made with these
	Wholemeal pasta, brown rice	White pasta, white rice
	Whole-grain breakfast cereals, e.g. Weetabix	Rice Krispies and corn flakes
	All-Bran, porridge, muesli and any cereals with added nuts and dried fruit	
	Whole-grain biscuits, e.g. digestives, flapjacks and cereal bars: biscuits containing nuts and dried fruit	Biscuits made from white flour, e.g. rich tea and wafers
	Whole-grain crackers, crispbreads, rye crispbreads, oatcakes	Crispbreads and crackers made from white flour, e.g. cream crackers

PRODUCT	NOT ALLOWED	ALLOWED
Fruit	All dried fruit, berries and bananas	All other fruit, maximum two portions a day; avoid skins, seeds and stalks
Vegetables	All pulses, beans, chickpeas, lentils, peas, sweet corn, Brussels sprouts	All other vegetables, maximum two portions a day in addition to potato; avoid skins, seeds and stalks
Miscellaneous	Nuts, seeds	Fruit and vegetable juices (not prune juice)

REINTRODUCING FIBRE

Week 1 - Try eating the skins on fruit and vegetables, e.g. apples, pears and cooked potatoes.

Week 2 – Eat an extra piece of fruit a day, e.g. a banana (not dried fruit) or an extra portion of vegetables (but not pulses). Five portions a day of fruit and vegetables (not including potatoes) are recommended long term for a healthy diet. Remember that one glass of fruit juice counts as one portion of fruit.

Week 3 – Try replacing white bread with wholemeal bread.

Week 4 – Try a higher fibre breakfast cereal such as Weetabix. Try Shredded Wheat or bran flakes.

Week 5 – If you are still symptom-free you may also like to try dried fruit or pulses.

Remember that these reintroductions provide a gradual build up of the amount of fibre in your diet. The aim is to identify a level of fibre that you can comfortably eat. You may find you can have high-fibre vegetables on days when you don't have wholemeal bread and high-fibre breakfast cereals, or vice versa. If so, try varying the sources of your fibre intake on a daily basis to achieve a balanced diet.

IgG Food Antibodies

It is not easy to follow an exclusion diet. Although the benefits are often spectacular, it nonetheless requires several weeks of determined self-control to determine accurately which foods upset you and must be avoided. Oh, for a simpler way forward! Enormous efforts have been made to find ways of determining which foods were culprits without the need for an exclusion diet. Some of these have verged on the ludicrous – such as holding a pendulum over the belly and seeing which way it swings – while others, such as skin testing, have been more logical but based on the false premise that these reactions are caused by some form of immuno-logical response to the foods.

As we now know that food intolerances in IBS are usually mediated by abnormal bacterial fermentation none of these methods can be reliable – and they are not! Nevertheless, recently much confusion and uncertainty have been caused because firms have marketed tests and devices that detect antibodies against foods that are not the usual allergy type (IgE) but of a different class – IgG. These IgG antibodies to foods certainly exist – they can be shown to be present in perfectly healthy blood-donors, and therefore probably do little harm.

Nevertheless, a study published in the prestigious British gastroenterological journal Gut *in 2004 reported a three-month trial in which 150 IBS patients received either a 'true' diet excluding all foods to which they had raised IgG antibodies, or a sham diet excluding the same number of foods but not those to which they had antibodies. At the end of the trial the true diet caused an overall 10 per cent greater reduction in symptoms than the sham diet, and there was a 26 per cent improvement in the case of patients who had kept carefully to their diets. Clearly the true diets were doing a lot of good.*

Why, then, do we not recommend our patients to have their IgG antibodies measured? There are three main reasons. First, we get better results with our low-fibre or exclusion diets. We know that approximately 70 per cent of our patients will get better, whereas the figure quoted for the IgG diet is 25–33 per cent. Second, we don't want our patients to avoid foods that don't really upset them. When we compared food intolerances in 20 IBS patients following a diet to the foods picked up by IgG antibody tests, the correlation was poor. Finally, IgG tests are expensive, and we believe this expense is not justified by the results. Spend your money on something more useful!

THE EXCLUSION DIET

If the recommendations we have made so far have not relieved your symptoms, now is the time to consider whether a specific food or group of foods is making your symptoms worse. An exclusion diet will help you to find out whether you have any specific food intolerances. It can be difficult to pinpoint individual foods because the ones that are most likely to upset you are the ones we tend to eat every day.

Although some foods are more likely to be responsible for IBS symptoms than others, the only way to decide which foods upset *you* is to test them individually. Excluding one food at a time may not be helpful if you have more than one food intolerance. For this reason a safe, simple diet, containing none of the common problem foods, needs to be followed for two weeks. If at the end of this you feel there has been a definite improvement in your symptoms, reintroduce the foods one at a time. If, however, you feel there has been little or no change, you should stop the exclusion diet and return to your normal eating.

A common problem in the first few days of the exclusion diet is that you may feel very much worse. Most patients lose a little weight, which may be a bonus. However, it's also common to develop severe headaches, tiredness, abdominal pain and aching in the limbs. The headaches have been suggested to be caused by withdrawal of coffee and tea but we have suggested that symptoms may also arise because of the death of many bacteria when deprived of their customary food sources, as the diet begins.

The breakdown of bacteria may release toxic chemicals contained within them (endotoxins), which make you feel dreadful. If this happens, do not despair. A reaction like this at the beginning of the diet nearly always means that the patient has genuine food intolerances and that the symptoms will clear in three to four days, when patients will feel much better. Make sure you drink plenty of liquids. Try to avoid taking painkillers if you can, but if necessary use a soluble preparation (such as soluble paracetamol or Solpadeine), as these do not contain any cereal starches.

GETTING STARTED

Before starting the exclusion diet, please discuss it with your doctor to ensure that he or she thinks this approach is sensible. You should also discuss whether or not to continue with any medication you may be taking. In general it's better to take as few pills as possible when trying an exclusion diet, as many contain starch and may be part of the problem.

You must consider how long it will take you to complete the diet and when would be the best time to start. The basic diet takes just two weeks, but if you improve, you will have to begin the gradual reintroduction of food and this may take two to three months, depending on how many foods cause problems. It may, for example, be better to delay starting until a holiday or busy social or work period is out of the way. We don't recommend that our patients start diets just before Christmas! Be prepared to make some sacrifices. In the early stages of the diet, for example, takeaways are not recommended.

THE EXCLUSION DIET

For the first two weeks of the exclusion diet, avoid all the foods in the 'not allowed' column and replace them with those on the 'allowed' column.

PRODUCT	NOT ALLOWED	ALLOWED
Meat	Beef, meat products, e.g. sausages, beef burgers, meat pies, paté	All other meat and poultry, e.g. chicken, turkey, lamb, pork (including ham and bacon), liver, kidney
Fish	Fish in batter or breadcrumbs or tinned in vegetable oil	All other fresh, smoked and tinned fish and shellfish
Vegetables	Potatoes, onion, sweetcorn, baked beans	Sweet potatoes and all other vegetables, including salad and pulses
Fruit	Citrus fruit, e.g. oranges, lemons, grapefruit	All other fruit, fresh, tinned and dried
Cereals	Wheat, oats, rye, corn, barley (check food labelling for these items)	Rice, rice cakes, ground rice, Rice Krispies, rice noodles, rice pasta, tapioca, sago and arrowroot
Cooking oils	Vegetable oils, corn oil (many foods contain corn oil: check labelling), nut oils	Sunflower, soya, olive, rapeseed, safflower oils
Dairy products	Cow's, goat's and sheep's milk and products, butter, margarine, cream, cheese, yoghurt, ice cream, eggs (check food labelling for these)	Soya milk and products, e.g. dairy-free margarine, tofu, soya yoghurt, soya cream and soya ice cream, sorbet (non-citrus): check labelling
Beverages	Tea, coffee (including decaffeinated), squashes and fizzy drinks, citrus fruit juice, alcohol, tap water	Herbal and fruit teas, Ribena, non-citrus fruit juices, e.g. apple, pineapple, tomato and mineral water
Miscellaneous	Yeast (check food labelling), salad cream and dressings, mustard, vinegar, tinned or packet sauces, chocolate, sweets and nuts	Salt, pepper, herbs, spices in moderation, sugar, honey, syrup, jam (non-citrus), carob, Kendal mint cake, seeds, e.g. sesame snaps, halva, tahini

FOLLOWING AN EXCLUSION DIET

Here are some pointers to help you through the diet:

➤ For two weeks before starting, record all the symptoms you have had (see pages 13, 42), and when. This will help assess the value of the diet later on.

➤ For the first two weeks of the exclusion diet keep strictly to the list of allowed foods on page 69. Remember that it is essential to continue for two weeks. All traces of offending foods eaten before the diet begins must disappear from the body before symptoms clear, so improvement is rarely seen in the first week. Don't give up. If you take a day off you will have wasted all your previous efforts, and will have to start again from the beginning.

➤ During the first fortnight, exclude any foods that you already suspect upset you as well as those listed on page 69. Later on, you will test and assess them properly.

➤ During the second week, eat as wide a variety of the 'allowed' foods as possible. This will help you to spot any unusual food intolerances.

➤ Throughout the two weeks, keep an accurate diary of everything you eat and drink, which symptoms you have, and when. Use a small notebook and allow a spread of two pages for each day.

If your symptoms have gone, proceed to the next stage of the diet – food reintroduction (page 71). If your symptoms have only partially improved, it may be helpful to continue the basic diet for just one further week, using your food and symptom diary (see page 42) to help spot any unusual food intolerances.

A sudden attack of pain or diarrhoea, for example, was probably provoked by something you ate the previous day. Start to reintroduce new foods only if there has been a clear improvement in your symptoms. If not, return to your normal diet.

If after two weeks your symptoms have not improved it is unlikely that food intolerance is the cause of your problems. Go back to normal eating and re-try the questionnaire in Chapter 3 to see if you may be suffering from a different form of IBS.

FOOD REINTRODUCTION

Hopefully you are now feeling delighted by the relief of your symptoms that the diet has brought. It's now very likely that your IBS can be controlled by diet. Nevertheless, to find out exactly which foods are responsible still requires very careful planning. Continue to keep your food and symptom diary throughout the phase of food reintroduction. The list on pages 74–75 shows the order in which we now recommend testing foods – based on our experience with many patients. Try to keep to the following rules when reintroducing foods:

➤ Reintroduce one food every two days until you have a reaction.

➤ Eat plenty of the foods you are testing (have at least two helpings daily or at least the amount specified in the reintroduction list). If on the morning after the last test day there are no ill effects, you may assume that the food is safe to eat and you can include it as normal in your basic diet.

➤ If you have a reaction, stop eating the food you are testing immediately. If you continue eating it, it will only make the symptoms worse. The time it takes to recover from a reaction varies. Do not test any new foods until you are completely well again, otherwise it will be difficult to tell if any symptoms that follow are due to the new food or left over from the food that previously upset you.

➤ Do not try to rush through the list of foods – the more haste, the less speed. The average reintroduction time is two months, but it may be longer if you react to several foods.

➤ The time it takes the symptoms to show also varies. Do not expect symptoms to develop immediately after eating a food, as happens with a food allergy. With food intolerance it may take 24 to 48 hours for a reaction to show. Sometimes symptoms appear so slowly that they are hardly noticeable to begin with. This is why it is important to keep a diary – you can look back and see when you were last really well and this should help you to spot the offending food.

➤ Drink plenty of water to help recover from a reaction. Some people find that adding a teaspoon of bicarbonate of soda in a glass of water increases the effectiveness of this treatment. If you need any painkillers, take only the soluble preparations of paracetamol (or Solpadeine).

➤ Some foods are made up of more than one ingredient. These ingredients will need to be tested separately. Otherwise, if a reaction occurs, you will not know which ingredient was to blame. Bread, for example, is made from yeast and wheat and you will need to test yeast first, before you can test the wheat in bread.

➤ Try to include foods in the order that they appear on pages 74–75. You may miss out a food that you never eat, but if it is included in an ingredient in another food that you do eat, then you should still test it. For example, you might not eat boiled or fried eggs, but you may eat a cake that is made with egg. Foods eaten only occasionally can be moved to the end of the list, but do not forget to test them.

➤ If, before starting the diet, you suspect that a particular food upsets you, you should still test it again anyway as you may have identified it wrongly.

➤ Take a week to test wheat as symptoms often develop slowly after this and may be missed. For the first four days, test white wheat products such as white flour, pasta and white bread (if yeast is tolerated). For the remaining three days try testing higher-fibre wheat products, such as wholemeal or granary bread, and cereals such as Weetabix or Shreddies. It is wise to leave the testing of wheat until late in the reintroductions, when you have a little experience under your belt.

➤ Sometimes you may suspect that food upsets you, but you are not sure. Don't waste time testing and retesting one food. Leave it out for a few weeks and come back to it later when your diet is less restricted. If you are female, it may be helpful to retest the food at a different stage of the menstrual cycle.

➤ At the end of the reintroduction, you must go back and retest all the foods that you believe affect you. Some suspected reactions may have been coincidental and there is no point in avoiding a food unless you really have to.

ORDER OF FOOD REINTRODUCTION

Test each food for two days. Test at least twice a day or as indicated below.

Tap water	Take throughout day
Potatoes	Baked, boiled, mashed (without dairy products)
Milk	450 ml spread throughout the day
Yeast	Three brewer's yeast tablets (one with each meal) or two teaspoons fresh yeast spread (e.g. Marmite, Vegemite) on rice cakes, each day
Tea	At least two cups per day
Rye	Ryvita or rye bread (check wheat free) – only test rye bread if yeast is tolerated
Beef	Example: cold slices at lunch and steak/roast/mince in the evening
Butter or margarine	Eat these spread on rice cakes or potato
Onions	Test both cooked and raw
Eggs	Test two per day
Oats	Test two helpings of porridge, oatcakes or flapjacks per day
Coffee	Test both coffee beans and instant coffee
Chocolate	Test plain or cocoa
Citrus fruits	Test oranges, grapefruit, satsumas, etc or juices
Corn	Test corn flakes, corn flour or sweetcorn
Cheese	Try 60 g (2 oz) twice a day
White wine	Test two glasses. If yeast is not tolerated, test spirits such as vodka or white rum

Yoghurt	Test two small cartons a day
Wheat	Test for seven days taking wheat at each meal (see note on page 73 on wheat testing)
Nuts	Try different varieties 60 g (2 oz) twice daily
Barley	Test barley flakes or pearl barley
Vinegar	Test on chips or in salad dressing twice daily

FREQUENTLY ASKED QUESTIONS

WILL MY DIET BE NUTRITIONALLY BALANCED?

With any luck you will need to avoid only one or two foods and you will find your diet reasonably straightforward. If you are avoiding a number of foods, or a few important ones such as milk or wheat, ask your doctor to refer you to a dietitian to check that your diet is nutritionally balanced and to get ideas on replacement foods.

Try to eat a wide range of your safe foods, rather then restricting yourself to a few. Check that you are following the guidelines for a balanced diet outlined on pages 77–78. If you are intolerant to milk/dairy products, you may not be getting enough calcium in your diet. Choose calcium-enriched soya milk and include non-dairy sources of calcium in your diet, such as tofu (soya bean curd), soya cheese, tinned fish (with bones), seeds, nuts, dried fruits, green vegetables, pulses and white bread. You may require a calcium supplement and these are available from chemists. Discuss this with your GP or dietitian.

If you are avoiding a number of foods, you may benefit from a multi-vitamin or multi-vitamin and mineral supplement such as Centrum, Sanatogen Gold or Forceval. Again, discuss with your GP or dietitian and don't forget to check if the supplement is free from any of the ingredients that upset you, such as wheat, yeast, corn or lactose. It's inadvisable to take large doses of individual vitamins and minerals as they are wasted if they exceed the amount required by the body and may even, in some cases, be toxic.

WILL I BE ABLE TO EAT THE FOODS THAT UPSET ME AGAIN?

A reliable way to rid people of their food intolerance has not yet been found, although in the future probiotic bacteria may help (see Chapter 9). As with testing for food intolerances, several methods to relieve them have been tried and may be recommended by alternative practitioners. These include administering small quantities of the food as drops under the tongue or as an injection into the skin (known as enzyme-potentiated desensitisation). Various drugs have also been tried. However, in our experience these have all produced disappointing results. For the present, while the intolerance continues, you will have to resign yourself to excluding the upsetting foods – as long as that seems preferable to suffering the symptoms that they cause.

However, many people find that after avoiding the food for several months, it no longer upsets them or they can eat it in small amounts and get away with very few ill effects. You should therefore recheck your food intolerances periodically – every six months – and you may be pleasantly surprised.

COULD I DEVELOP MORE FOOD INTOLERANCES?

Intolerances can change. They can disappear and, occasionally, new ones can develop. Surgery, antibiotics, virus infections and bouts of gastroenteritis (food poisoning) are some of the reasons for this happening. It may be easy to identify a food that has brought back your symptoms, but if not, you will need to take yourself through the basic two-week diet and food testing again.

WHAT SHOULD I DO IF I HAVE SEVERAL FOOD INTOLERANCES?

We have found that patients with IBS rarely have multiple food intolerances. However, if you are unlucky and find that a large number of foods upset you, you should think seriously about whether it is worth trying to control your symptoms by diet. It may be that you should avoid foods that cause the worst effects and try to control the remaining symptoms in other ways. You should certainly ask your GP to refer you to a dietitian who can check the nutritional value of what you are eating and you should discuss other ways of coping with your symptoms with your doctor. If it's agreed that you can safely continue controlling your symptoms by diet rather than with drugs, it may help if you rotate your diet.

Details of how to do this and suggestions as to sources of unusual foods which may be less likely to upset you are given in our previous book *Solve your Food Intolerances*, which is listed under 'further reading'. This book also contains many tempting recipes that we hope may persuade you that following an exclusion diet doesn't have to mean that your food is not exciting!

A SAMPLE MENU

The simple guidelines below are intended to help make sure that the exclusion diet you are following is nutritionally balanced.

Breakfast
➤ Rice Krispies, soya milk and sugar
➤ Rice cakes, milk-free margarine and jam
➤ Apple juice/herbal tea

Snacks
➤ Meat/poultry/fish
➤ Cold rice salad or rice cakes
➤ Salad
➤ Fruit/soya yoghurt
➤ Ribena

Main meal
➤ Meat/poultry/fish
➤ Sweet potato/rice/buckwheat pasta/rice noodles
➤ Vegetables
➤ Fruit
➤ Soya-based dessert
➤ Herbal tea

LOW-FIBRE, GLUTEN-FREE DIET

Gluten is the protein found in wheat and some other cereals. Following a gluten-free diet involves avoiding wheat, rye and barley. Oats, used in porridge, oatcakes, and flapjacks, are high in fibre and contain a similar protein to gluten called avenin.

Coeliac Disease

There is much confusion among patients and some doctors between wheat intolerance and coeliac disease. Coeliac disease is caused by a reaction between gluten in cereals and the body's immune system. The lining of the small intestine is damaged and food cannot be absorbed properly, leading to failure to thrive, anaemia and bone disease. If gluten is withdrawn from the diet, patients make a speedy recovery.

This is quite different from the wheat intolerance of IBS, where it is believed that bacterial breakdown of wheat leads to the production of toxic chemicals and the small intestine is quite normal. Nevertheless, coeliac disease must be excluded before starting any patient on a gluten-free diet. Formerly, it was necessary to take a biopsy (tissue sample) of the lining of the small bowel for this purpose, but nowadays it is a simple matter to take a blood test. This measures levels of the enzyme transglutaminase, which breaks down gluten in such a way as to trigger the immune response. It is important that you do not have this test done whilst you are on a gluten-free diet as its accuracy depends on you continuing to eat gluten.

You will need to study food labels to see which foods contain gluten. Wheat, rye, oats and barley will be listed in the ingredients list if these are included in the product. By law, food labels must say if food contains gluten from wheat, rye, oats, barley, spelt, kamut and their hybridised strains. Some manufacturers also use the crossed-grain symbol to indicate whether a product is gluten-free, but this is not a legal requirement.

There are many specially manufactured gluten-free products available on the market. Initially these were developed for people with coeliac disease. Some of the specially manufactured gluten-free foods contain gluten-free wheat starch. This is where the gluten has been chemically separated from wheat starch, making the product suitable for inclusion in a gluten-free diet.

Some foods that are gluten-free are not low in fibre, so you will need to consider whether the food is both gluten -free and low in fibre. The fibre content of the food may be listed on the nutritional labelling, per 100 g of product and per typical portion size. This information must be present if the product makes a health claim, such as 'low fat' or 'high fibre'. A product may have a high content of fibre per 100 g, though the portion size consumed may be small, making the overall fibre content low. Gluten-free fibre and multigrain seeded breads have a high-fibre content. Not all gluten-free white breads are low in fibre, probably due to the guar gum, xantham gum and powdered cellulose that are added to improve the textures of the breads.

Quite a lot to think about before starting the diet, though the diet sheet below should guide you.

LOW-FIBRE GLUTEN-FREE INFORMATION SHEET

FOODS GROUPS	LOW IN FIBRE AND GLUTEN-FREE	NEED TO CHECK	FOODS TO AVOID, DUE TO THEIR HIGH FIBRE OR GLUTEN CONTENT
Meat	Fresh meat and poultry, bacon, smoked meats, cured pure meats, parma ham	Burgers, ham, sausages	Meat and poultry cooked in batter or breadcrumbs, faggots, rissoles, haggis, breaded ham
Fish	All fresh fish and shellfish, smoked, kippered and dried fish, fish canned in oil or brine	Fish in sauce, fish pastes and pâtés	Fish in batter or breadcrumbs, fish cakes, taramasalata, fish fingers

Dairy products	Fresh, UHT, dried, condensed, evaporated, goat's and sheep's milk, fresh and soured cream, buttermilk, crème fraîche, cheese and eggs	Yoghurt, fromage frais, soya milk	Milk with added fibre, oat milk, yoghurt and fromage frais containing muesli or cereals, scotch eggs, cheese containing beer, Christmas cake
Cereals and flour	Corn, cornflour, cornmeal, white rice, arrowroot, tapioca, sago, cassava, polenta, corn tortillas		Wheat, bulgar wheat, durum wheat, wheat bran, wheatgerm, wheat starch, semolina, cous cous, barley, malt, malted barley, rye, triticale, spelt, quinoa, amaranth, buckwheat, millet, gram flour, soya flour, potato flour
Bread, cakes and biscuits	Gluten-free white flour and products made with gluten-free white flour, gluten-free pizza bases		Ordinary bread, biscuits, cakes, pastries, scones, muffins and pizza, rye crispbreads, oat cakes, multi-grain seeded loaves
Pasta and noodles	Corn pasta, rice pasta		Fresh, dried and canned wheat pasta, noodles, buckwheat pasta, rice and millet pasta
Breakfast cereals	Rice Krispies	Malted breakfast cereals	Wheat-based breakfast cereals, muesli, oats, puffed rice cereals, rice and millet cereals, gluten-free cereals with added dried fruits and nuts
Fats and oils	Butter, margarine, cooking oils	Suet	

Nuts, seeds and pulses			Nuts, peanut butter, seeds, pulse-type beans, e.g. baked, broad, butter, kidney, chick peas, lentils
Savoury snacks	Home-made popcorn		Crisps, snacks made from wheat, rye, barley and oats, pretzels
Preserves and spreads	Honey, syrup, jam, marmalade (avoid pips/seeds)	Lemon curd	Mincemeat
Soups, sauces, pickles and seasonings	Tomato and garlic purée, herbs and spices, vinegars, ground pepper, mint sauces, tamari	Gravy granules, stock cubes, soups other than those listed as being high in fibre , packet and sauces in jars, mustard, mayonnaise, salad cream, dressings, Worcestershire sauce, soya desserts	Soy sauce, stuffing mix, pickles and chutneys lentil, pea and bean soups
Confectionery and puddings	Jelly, sorbets, milk puddings made with gluten-free ingredients, boiled sweets	Sweets, chocolates, chewing gum, ice cream and lollies, custard powder, mousse	Confectionery containing fruit and nuts, puddings made using wheat flour
Drinks	Tea, coffee, fruit juice, squash, clear fizzy drinks, cocoa, wine, spirits, cider, sherry, port, liqueurs, gluten-free beers	Drinking chocolate, tomato juice	Malted milk drinks, barley waters, cloudy fizzy drinks, vending machine hot chocolate, beer, lager, ales, stout
Miscellaneous	Gelatine, bicarbonate of soda, cream of tartar, fresh and dried yeast, artificial sweeteners, Bovril, Marmite, icing sugar	Tofu, cake decorations, baking powder	Marzipan, ice cream cones and wafers, liquorice

Fruit Where possible avoid skins and seeds. Keep to a maximum of 2 portions a day.	Apples Apricot Cherries Fruit cocktail Grapefruit Grapes Kiwi Lychees Mango Nectarine Oranges Peaches Pears Pineapple Plums Rhubarb Satsumas Strawberries Tangerines		Dried Fruit Banana chips Bananas Blackberries Cranberries Currants Dates, figs Gooseberries Loganberries Prunes Raisins Raspberrries Redcurrants Sultanas
Vegetables Where possible avoid skins, seeds and stalks. Keep to a maximum of 2 portions a day in addition to potato	Asparagus Aubergine Beetroot Carrot Celery Courgette Cucumber Leeks Lettuce Marrow Mushroom Onion Pepper Hot potato Radish Swede Tomato	Beansprouts Green/French/ Runner Beans. Broccoli florets Cabbage Cauliflower florets Mange-tout Parsnips Spinach Spring greens Sweet potato (These vegetables have a moderate fibre content. Allow small portions occasionally)	Pulse-type beans, eg baked, broad, butter, kidney. Brussel sprouts Chick peas Lentils Peas Sweetcorn.

The low-fibre gluten-free diet should be followed for a month to assess its value. If no improvement has then occurred, you should go back to normal eating. If you feel better, you must try to decide whether it is the low-fibre foods that are helping or whether you are truly upset by gluten. This may be done as follows:

Week 1 – Try eating skins on fruits and vegetables.
Week 2 – Try an extra piece of fruit per day, e.g. a banana or extra portion of vegetables.
Week 3 – Introduce wheat as white pasta.
Week 4 – If white pasta causes no ill effects, try wholemeal bread.

If any food item brings back your symptoms you should then, of course, avoid it.

Candida and IBS

An American physician, Dr C. Orion Truss, suggested that IBS symptoms are caused by a yeast called Candida albicans. Infections by Candida are very common. The most frequent are infections of the vagina ('thrush') and infections in the mouth in children. Dr Truss suggested that overgrowth of Candida in the gut might be an important factor in the development of IBS. He developed a diet low in sugar, yeast and mould-containing foods. These foods were avoided because they were thought likely to promote the growth of fungi such as Candida. This diet relieved many of the patients' symptoms.

His theory has been taken up enthusiastically by many practitioners of alternative or complementary medicine who diagnose gastrointestinal candida on the basis of a range of symptoms including chronic fatigue, poor concentration, impaired memory, pain in muscles and joints, skin problems and urinary difficulties together with the IBS symptoms. They are treated with a combination of Dr Truss' diet and antifungal drugs and many improve.

We are very sceptical of the importance of Candida in IBS. Candida is present in the gut flora of all normal individuals and vaginal thrush is very common in women who have never had any difficulties with IBS at all. Moreover, Candida can be treated by specific anti-fungal drugs alone. We examined stools from 40 food-intolerant IBS patients and the same number of normal healthy people and found absolutely no difference in the numbers of Candida present between both groups.

Why, then, did Dr Truss' patients improve? We believe that this is because his anti-fungal diet is in fact very similar to our exclusion diet. Major items such as cereals, dairy products and yeasts are all excluded and thus this diet can be expected to influence bacterial metabolism in just the same way as our diet has been shown to do. If Candida were the root of the problem, Dr Truss' patients should have benefited from anti-fungal drugs alone. In a study performed on a group of women suffering from vaginal thrush as well as the associating symptoms of candida, there was no effect of combined oral and vaginal treatment with an anti-fungal drug that is highly effective in clearing up Candida infections. These women did not alter their diets, proving that the drug alone was ineffective.

SUMMARY

➤ Malfermentation may be caused by the action of certain types of gut bacteria on the fibre in food.

➤ Other causes include intolerance to certain foods, especially to gluten-containing cereals, dairy products, eggs, yeast, onions, potatoes, chocolate and beverages.

➤ Malfermentation can be treated by low-fibre, gluten-free diets and by an exclusion diet.

➤ Try the low-fibre diet first and, if symptoms improve, slowly reintroduce fibre into your diet until you find a level you can tolerate.

➤ If a low-fibre diet does not help, try an exclusion diet by eating only 'safe' foods (see page 69) for two weeks and then reintroducing other foods one by one until you find which ones cause symptoms.

➤ If you react badly to several foods, ask your doctor to refer you to a dietitian for advice.

➤ If wheat products are causing symptoms, combine a gluten-free diet with a low-fibre diet and then try to determine whether fibre or gluten is the cause of your problem.

CHAPTER 6

Overload and Overflow

If you scored highly for overload and overflow in the questionnaire on page 39 then this chapter is the way forward for you. Overload and overflow is an important cause of IBS, responsible for up to 20 per cent of cases. Patients with this problem report intermittent bouts of painful diarrhoea occurring at intervals of seven to 14 days. In between these bouts they believe that their motions are normal, as they pass a formed stool most days. However, these stools are usually small (Types 1 and 2 on the Bristol Stool Form Scale – see page 26) and this shows the bowel is not being adequately emptied each day. Therefore, the amount of faeces remaining builds up until finally it reaches a critical threshold, at which stage various trigger factors can cause a sudden and often urgent bout of diarrhoea. Rich meals are an important trigger and stress is another. If the problem is correctly treated, however, neither of these factors have any effect on the bowels.

Sometimes severe constipation can lead to overflow diarrhoea. This seems particularly common in elderly people when faeces becomes impacted in the bowel. The whole rectum then becomes stuffed with faeces that is too hard or too painful to expel. This can lead to 'spurious diarrhoea', in which liquid material flows past the impacted material in the rectum and leaks out, causing incontinence.

Our patients with overload and overflow did not have faecal impaction because, on examination, their rectums were always empty. However, when we examined their abdomens it was quite easy to feel the large bowel. This is not usually possible in normal individuals. We found that the bowel could be felt in 60 per cent of cases of simple constipation and 60 per cent of cases of overload and overflow.

In comparison, it could be felt in only 13 per cent of those with anxiety, or food intolerance. Thus patients with overload and overflow seem to have an excess of faeces in their bowel, which at a critical stage became liable to be expelled rapidly leading to pain and diarrhoea. The hallmark of this condition is intermittent diarrhoea with an easy-to-feel loaded colon.

If the bowel is overloaded, the logical approach is to empty it. One of the most valuable techniques in modern gastroenterology is colonoscopy. This is often carried out in patients with IBS to exclude more serious disease. Here, an endoscope (flexible viewing tube) is passed through the anus and along the large intestine to search for polyps, cancer or inflammation. To perform this examination successfully the bowel must be empty and this requires powerful purges using medication such as Picolax.

Patients often commented on how much better they felt after a bowel clear-out of this sort, and we wondered if the improvement might persist if we kept the bowel from becoming overloaded again. We started to treat these patients with bulk laxatives such as sterculia (Normacol) and linseed – non-fermentable fibre – to speed the passage of stools along the bowel so that a larger volume of stools were expelled daily and over-loading no longer occurred. This was what happened. We went on to do a formal study with 15 patients and found that six months later 12 were still completely well, with no further IBS problems.

GETTING STARTED

The first stage is to empty the bowel completely. It is no good going onto bulk laxatives if the bowel is already overloaded as they will only make you feel more bloated and uncomfortable. Don't start any bulk laxatives until the day after the bowel clearout has been performed.

➤ Choose a suitable day for your bowel clearout. Purges such as Picolax, Citramag and Movicol will make you go to the lavatory very frequently. Choose a day when you don't need to go to work or out shopping and can stay at home. A weekend is often ideal for this purpose.

➤ Choose which purge you are going to use. You may like to discuss this with your GP. They are very concentrated solutions and they therefore sometimes cause nausea, bloating and even vomiting and, less frequently, abdominal cramps, which normally settle fairly quickly. **You should not take bowel cleansing solutions if you are pregnant or have heart or kidney disease or diabetes.**

➤ Picolax: follow the patient information leaflet carefully on making and taking the solution. Heat is generated when Picolax is added to water. For this reason the powder should be added initially to two tablespoons of water (30 ml). After five minutes, when the heat reaction and production is complete, the solution should be further diluted to a tumbler-full (150 ml) of water before being consumed. One sachet is taken in the morning before 8am and a second in the afternoon between 2pm and 4pm. It acts within three hours of the first dose. On the same day you should drink copious amounts of water or another chosen clear fluid, to flush the system through. We recommend one large glass (600 ml) of water every hour.

➤ Citramag: again, follow the patient information leaflet carefully on making and taking the solution. Each sachet is dissolved in 200 mls of hot water. The first is taken at 8am and the second between 2pm and 4pm. Like Picolax, it is necessary to take copious amounts of clear fluid during the day, again one large glass (600 ml) every hour.

➤ Movicol (polyethylene glycol): dissolve eight sachets in 1 litre of water and drink over the next six hours. This is somewhat milder than Picolax or Citramag, but just as effective. **Patients with heart disease should be careful when taking this, however, so consult your doctor first.**

➤ Two other powerful bowel cleansing agents that are available are Fleet Phospho-soda and Klean-Prep. We don't recommend either of these. Fleet is very powerful. However, such a high degree of cleansing, although fine for colonoscopy, is not always necessary for the treatment of overflow and overload and can occasionally produce ulcers in the bowel. As for Kleen-prep, it's necessary to drink a tumbler-full of the solution every 10 to 15 minutes until 4 litres (6 ½ pints) have been taken. Such a large amount of fluid can be difficult for some patients to cope with.

WHAT HAPPENS NEXT?

These bowel cleansing agents produce an initial bout of diarrhoea that dies away in three to four hours after the second dose. This should leave you feeling very much more comfortable. The following morning you should start your bulk laxatives to keep the bowels ticking over smoothly. **Use an agent that cannot be broken down by the bowel bacteria,** otherwise this may lead to the production of excess wind, bloating and even diarrhoea. In particular, **avoid** laxatives based on ispaghula husk and check the label of specific products. Herbalists sometimes recommend Psyllium. This is made from the same husk and again is not ideal for this purpose. **Avoid wheat bran and other cereal products.**

You may like to discuss with your GP which bulk-forming laxative you use, although these are all available over the counter, so it is not necessary to get a prescription. Ones available are:

➤ Methyl cellulose: a dose of this is three to six tablets twice daily. Those should be well-chewed and taken with at least 300 mls of liquid. Experiment with the dose so that you get a bulky soft stool daily that is easy to pass without straining.

➤ Sterculia (Normacol): this comes as granules (usually in 7 g sachets). Dose is one to three heaped teaspoons taken once or twice daily after meals and washed down with plenty of water. Putting the granules into water forms a sludge that is difficult to swallow and lingers in the mouth. We have found that it is easier to mix the granules into yoghurt, which makes the granules go down without difficulty, or a fizzy drink, which keeps the granules in suspension so that they may be swallowed without difficulty. (*There is another form of Normacol available called Normacol Plus. This contains a stimulant laxative, frangula, as well as the sterculia and* **we don't recommend** *taking this on a daily basis.*)

➤ Linseed is available from health food stores. The normal dose is two to four tablespoons daily. This can easily be sprinkled on to cereals or soups. This must be followed by a full glass of water.

These bulk-forming laxatives swell in liquid **and should not be taken immediately before going to bed**. We advise that a second dose, if necessary, is taken before 6pm in the evening. However, these products are very safe. Clearly if you take too much you may find you are going to the loo more frequently than you wish. If this happens, reduce the dose. Experiment with different doses to find which give you the most comfortable and easily passed motion.

WHAT HAPPENS IN THE LONG TERM?

If the bulk laxative dose is correct, you should pass regular stools that prevent the large intestine becoming overloaded with faeces. This will keep you comfortable and attacks of diarrhoea and pain will not occur. Remember to take plenty of fluid with your laxatives – at least a large tumbler-full after each dose, on top of your normal fluid intake.

Some patients remain completely comfortable and have no need for further treatment. Others find that after a while the bulk laxative appears to lose some of its effectiveness and they detect signs that the bowel is once again showing signs of becoming overloaded. Their stools may become smaller and harder to pass and they develop abdominal bloating and discomfort.

If this happens, you should take a dose of a stimulant laxative, such as a single dose of two to four Senokot tablets, or one or two Bisacodyl tablets, at night, as well as the bulk-forming laxative. This should be enough to empty the bowel and get everything running smoothly again. It may be necessary to take a repeat dose of this kind every so often. If this starts to happen more regularly than weekly, you should seek advice from your GP. It's not usually necessary to go back to Picolax, Citramag or Movicol.

Another problem sometimes encountered is that patients still have excess wind. If this happens it may be sensible to combine the bulk laxative with a low-fibre diet, as fermentable fibre often gives rise to excess gas and it is this that causes your bloating. Thus a combination of the low-fibre diet and non-fermenting, bulk-forming laxatives can provide all the health benefits of fibre in the diet, while at the same time avoiding gas and flatulence.

We don't know the cause of overload and overflow IBS. However, some patients do have gluten intolerance as well, so if the low-fibre diet on top of the bulk-forming laxative is not sufficient to control any remaining symptoms, it may be worth a two-week trial of a low-fibre gluten-free diet (see page 78) while at the same time continuing with the non-fermentable bulk laxative.

Joggers' Diarrhoea

Sometimes athletes suffer diarrhoea after a run. The Medical Officer in charge of the London Marathon has told us that this is a fairly common problem, and causes a number of runners to fall out each year. Sometimes the problem is abdominal pain rather than diarrhoea, perhaps during the evening after the race. When this is investigated, no abnormality can be discovered, so this problem falls within the definition of IBS.

The major difference from other forms of IBS is that the attacks are not triggered by eating, nor by stress – but only by running. We performed a study to see if there was any evidence that exercise lead to malfermentation in healthy runners – but no increase in hydrogen excretion occurred.

It's now believed that joggers' diarrhoea is caused by the blood supply to the gut being insufficient during exercise. When we run, more blood must be diverted to the muscles to meet the great increase in demand for oxygen and nutrients which then occurs. The amount of blood flowing to the brain, heart and kidneys is kept constant, come what may, because a reduction in blood supply to these organs can be dangerous. The result is that the amount of blood available for the gut may be reduced. If it falls below a certain level, abdominal pain and diarrhoea may result.

Joggers' diarrhoea is, therefore, a sign that the athlete is not fit enough. When we train and become fitter, the heart is able to pump more blood, ensuring that an adequate supply is available for all our organs – gut included. The solution is to slow down, and reduce the amount of effort we demand of our bodies. This, of course, relieves the attacks of diarrhoea. The next step is slowly and gradually to build up our fitness over a matter of weeks so that we find that we are later able to run the required distances at the required speed – but without suffering any abdominal problems!

SUMMARY

➤ Overload and overflow is due to a build-up of faeces in the bowel that becomes impacted. Some faeces leaks out, causing diarrhoea. The cause is not known.

➤ Treatment is to use a bowel cleansing solution to clear out the bowel and then to use a non-fermenting bulk laxative to prevent the faeces becoming impacted again.

➤ Do not take bowel cleansing solutions if you are pregnant or have heart or kidney disease or diabetes.

➤ See a doctor first if you have any other on-going medical condition.

➤ Use only the bowel cleansing solutions and laxatives recommended (see pages 89–91) as some types are too powerful or have unpleasant side effects.

➤ If excess wind and bloating are a problem, combine this treatment with a low-fibre diet – see page 78.

CHAPTER 7

Air Swallowing and Anxiety

Most of us swallow a little air with every mouthful of food we eat. This air can usually easily be absorbed from the stomach into the bloodstream and into the lungs. Trouble may arise, however, if we swallow too much air. Air can collect in the stomach and produce a number of ill effects. The stomach may become distended, which in itself may cause discomfort under the ribs on the left. Frequently the fullness caused by this distension causes people to feel that the stomach is full up, even though they have not eaten a proper meal.

Air coming back up will lead to belching and sometimes to acid reflux or even vomiting. Some of the air may leave the stomach via the duodenum and pass along the small intestine. This too may cause pain by distending the gut. As the air passes along the bowel it may produce rumblings and uncomfortable bloating. Finally, it will pass out through the anus causing embarrassing wind. Air swallowing of this sort is an important cause of IBS.

WHY DO WE SWALLOW AIR?

Excess air swallowing may arise for a number of reasons, including heartburn, hiatus hernia and a blocked nose (see page 108), but anxiety is perhaps the most common cause. Anxious IBS patients often develop an abnormal form of rapid yet shallow breathing known as over-breathing, hyperventilation, or breathing pattern disorder (BPD). Normal breathing mainly involves the diaphragm, the sheet of muscle at the top of the abdomen, directly underneath the lungs. This is known as abdominal breathing and draws air through the nose and deep into the lungs. Abnormal breathing mostly involves the muscles of the upper chest, and involves rapid, shallow breathing using the mouth. This increases the amount of air going down the gullet into the stomach, causing excess wind, belching, bloating, rumbling and pain. A major cause of abnormal breathing is anxiety. Later on we explain how to manage anxiety. But first, how do you tell if your breathing pattern is abnormal?

TEST FOR ABNORMAL BREATHING PATTERNS

If you scored positive for anxiety and air swallowing on the questionnaire, this will have given you some insight into the problem. If your family and friends notice that you yawn and sigh frequently, this is often a strong pointer to abnormal breathing patterns. But to confirm it, you should do the following test:

1. Sit in front of a long mirror and place one hand on your abdomen between breastbone and navel.

2. Put the other hand on your breastbone just below the collar bones.

3. Take a deep breath and check for three things:

    ➤ Which part of your chest moved first?

    ➤ Which part of your chest moved the most?

    ➤ Did you breathe in with your nose or your mouth?

The natural breathing pattern is to breathe in through the nose and to see that your stomach expanded first with little if any movement of the hand resting on your upper chest. Someone with a breathing pattern disorder will breathe in fast, possibly through the mouth, the upper chest will expand first and there is little or no abdominal breathing – indeed the abdomen may have been sucked in. If you fall into this second group it is well worthwhile trying to correct your breathing habits as it's very likely that if you succeed, you are going to feel very much better.

HOW TO CORRECT ABNORMAL BREATHING PATTERN

Restoring a normal breathing pattern takes patience and a lot of concentration. Regular daily practice is essential. While some people learn quickly and are soon able to get back to normal breathing patterns, others may have to practise for months and may not be free from symptoms or setbacks for a whole year.

Starting to retrain your breathing may be uncomfortable at first, but using a conscious effort to restore a natural breathing pattern enables the respiratory centre in the brain, which controls breathing, to reset itself to balance the gases at the optimum level. The four basic principals of breathing retraining are:

1. Becoming aware of healthy breathing patterns and the need for change.

2. Learning slow nose breathing with the diaphragm.

3. Learning to relax the upper chest and shoulders.

4. Restoring normal breathing rates and volumes.

It is not easy to do this all by yourself and if you are able to have some sessions with a physiotherapist who specialises in breathing retraining you will find that this is extremely valuable. In Britain such expertise is not easy to find, but therapists working in this field are listed at www.physiohypervent.org.

Mrs Ann Copping, a retired physiotherapist specialising in breathing disorders with many years experience in this field, has prepared a DVD that not only explains the techniques but also provides invaluable demonstrations of the right way forward. (For details see Further Information page 194.)

GETTING STARTED

The following exercises were developed at Papworth Hospital by Dr Claude Lum and his physiotherapy team. They need to be practised regularly and for a considerable period of time if they are to be successful. Progress initially will vary but the good days should gradually get more frequent and the bad days less so. Monitor yourself on a monthly basis so that you get a better picture of what is happening.

EXERCISES IN WEEK ONE

1. Get into a comfortable position, for example, propped up slightly on your bed. If you have a comfortable armchair with a high back that can support your neck and shoulders you can use that.

2. Before you think about the breathing exercises make sure your shoulders are in a relaxed position. They should be as low as possible rather than elevated towards your ears.

3. Place one hand over your upper chest and one just above your pelvis. As you breathe in, try to push out your lower hand gently and to keep your top hand absolutely still. As you breathe out, just relax. The size of the breath should be what feels to be normal. The idea is to breathe as low down as possible, using the diaphragm, but not to take huge breaths. Practise this for a little while until you are happy with it – having lots of breaks, if necessary.

4. When you are happy with the position of your breathing you will need to think about its speed. This time, breathe in under your bottom hand, again keeping your top hand still, and then breathe straight out. Pause for two to three seconds before you breathe in again.

So the breathing pattern looks rather like this:

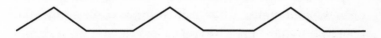

Breathe in. Breathe out. Pause for two to three seconds.

When you first do this you may feel 'air-hungry' – desperate to take a whole series of very rapid breaths. Don't despair. When you feel very uncomfortable, stop and have a rest. With time and practice, it will become easier and after a few days you will be able to manage the exercise for several minutes without having to have a break. To get the correct timing it might help if you count mentally: 1, 2 (*breathe in*), 3, 4 (*breathe out*), 5, 6, 7 (*relax*). Alternatively, you may wish to substitute a phrase containing seven syllables such as 'Tetley's...' (*breathe in*) '...Yorkshire...' (*breathe out*) '...Tea tastes great...' (*relax*). You may prefer to think up a seven syllable phrase of your own!

If you feel dizzy while you are doing this, you may be taking breaths that are too big rather than too deep. You can get over this dizziness by cupping both your hands over mouth and nose and re-breathing the air you breathe out for five or six slow breaths. This air contains more carbon dioxide (CO_2) than ordinary room air, and thus will increase the level of CO_2 in your blood. It is the CO_2 in blood, not the oxygen, that helps regulate your breathing. Continue doing this until the dizziness has gone.

Some patients have found that saying, 'Lips together, jaw relaxed, breathing low and slow', works for them. It may also help you to improve abdominal breathing by imagining that you are trying to expand your belt or an imaginary strip of elastic round your waist. To ensure that you are indeed moving your belly rather than your chest, check the movements with your hands, as described.

This is the basic exercise – breathe in gently with your diaphragm, breathe out, pause. You need to do this exercise four times a day for 10 minutes at a time and count how many breaths you do in one minute. The aim is to get down to between eight and 10 breaths per minute. Do not do any more than four 10-minute sessions in the first week.

EXERCISES IN WEEK TWO

Continue with the four 10-minute sessions you were doing in the first week. Into one of these sessions it is advisable to include some relaxation exercises (see below). Now try the slow diaphragmatic breathing exercise in the sitting position.

1. Sit comfortably with your back supported and check that your shoulders are not pushed up by the arms of

the chair. Practise this little and often during the day, trying to incorporate it into your routine activities such as watching television, sitting in a traffic jam or on a train or bus journey.

2. Next, try the exercise in the standing position also. This is harder because you need your abdominal muscles to work to stop you falling over, making it more difficult to relax. What is more, your diaphragm has to push against those contracted abdominal muscles. The key is to relax when you breathe out and not be tempted to suck your stomach back in. Forget the vanity! Again, practise this little and often during the day, perhaps while waiting for the kettle to boil or in a supermarket queue. In all these stationary positions you are aiming to breathe at eight to 10 breaths per minute.

EXERCISES IN WEEK THREE

Continue with all the previous exercises but now add in some breathing practice when you are moving around. It still must be low, diaphragmatic breathing but now it is not necessary to breathe quite so slowly, as exercise makes your body produce more CO_2. Start off practising when you are walking and then try the exercises while climbing the stairs. If you are moving quickly you need not put the pause into the breathing pattern.

After energetic exercise, we all breathe rapidly through our mouths in order to get in enough oxygen for the extra muscular activity. It is important, once exercise is over, that you revert back to correct nose breathing using the abdominal muscles as quickly as possible. After exercise, when your body slows down, try to consciously slow down your breathing too. Do it gradually but aim to get the breathing back to eight to 10 breaths per minute as soon as you can. Continue with these exercises regularly and soon the diaphragmatic breathing will become easier and more automatic.

If you have been accustomed to many months of mouth and upper chest breathing, this new method of breathing through your nose and into your belly will feel strange. You may feel short of breath, but this is a good sign showing you are making progress. If you feel breathless, STOP and check the position of your upper chest. Then relax not only your shoulders and upper chest, but all the muscles of the body. Focus on slow nose breathing. This routine has been described by some physiotherapists as STOP-DROP-FLOP.

COMMON DIFFICULTIES

Your diaphragm may be a little weak at first if it has been out of action for a long time. It may need strengthening. If you find yourself breathing in a jerky fashion, then it may help to place a moderate weight of 1.4–1.8 kg (3–4 lb) on your abdomen just below your tummy button while lying down. One patient found that her iron (switched off!) was just the right weight. If you have problems with heartburn lie in a semi-recumbent position.

People who suffer from asthma may need to pay special attention to their breathing after a wheezing attack. Breathing is usually chaotic during the attack, switching from upper to lower chest with little chance of control because there is an increased respiratory drive. The STOP-DROP-FLOP routine helps to reduce stress and fear while waiting for the asthma medication to work. Once the attack is over, re-establishing the nose breathing and relaxation of the upper chest must be the top priority.

Sometimes the urge to sigh, yawn or gulp air will at times seem overwhelming and uncomfortable. This is a sign of progress, however, and you should resist the temptation. With regular and determined practice, you will maintain your low volume nose breathing and the respiratory centres will get accustomed to the normal level of CO_2 in your blood, making you feel much more comfortable. Avoid tight-fitting clothes that may constrict your abdomen and stop you breathing properly with your diaphragm.

TALKING

Many people swallow air while speaking, particularly when they are excited and enjoying themselves, sometimes leading to agonising gut pains. So it is important to be aware of breathing patterns when you are talking. People with breathing pattern disorder tend to gulp in an enormous breath of air when starting to speak, and then gabble rapidly in long sentences. At the end of a sentence another great chestful of air is taken. Concentrate on speaking more slowly and on taking in sips of air during the sentence, breathing at commas as well as at full stops! This can be practised by reading out loud, particularly poetry, which usually has a rhythm that often shows the places where a breath should be taken.

Low Blood Sugar

Dr Lum believed that low blood sugar can play a part in attacks of anxiety and abnormal breathing. This condition, called reactive hypoglycaemia, is a controversial topic. Patients affected complain of a range of symptoms such as flushing, sweating, hunger,

---

headache, palpitations and shaking which come on shortly after eating foods containing sugar. When we eat sugar, the hormone insulin is rapidly released from the pancreas. In some cases of reactive hypoglycaemia there is increased sensitivity to insulin that then works so fast that the level of sugar in the blood falls too low, producing these symptoms. In other patients, however, the sugar level is found to be normal when these attacks occur, and so doctors have blamed it all on psychological causes.

Many of the symptoms of disordered breathing are, of course, related to anxiety and therefore psychological in origin, and Dr Lum taught that the true problem was the breathing disorder, rather than the precise level of the blood sugar. As the blood sugar falls, anxiety sets in, even before the sugar falls to abnormal levels. The anxiety sets off the abnormal breathing, and the attack begins.

As breathing re-training proceeds, of course, these attacks will become less severe. Nevertheless, Dr Lum urged his patients to avoid refined sugars, which cause rapid insulin release, and to prevent the blood sugar falling by eating snacks between meals of foods that were digested slowly. These produce a slow and prolonged increase in the level of sugar absorbed into the body and so prevent excess insulin production. These foods include complex carbohydrates such as Granary bread and whole-grain pasta, and proteins such as cheese, meat and egg. All will release sugar slowly, maintaining normal levels in the blood.

These foods are, of course, those that are recommended in a 'low-GI diet'. Much has recently appeared in the press about the health value of eating foods with a low glycaemic index – that is, foods which release sugar slowly into the blood. Such a diet helps prevent obesity and diabetes, and much else besides. Unfortunately, low-GI foods are also among those that are most likely to produce food intolerance, and for precisely the same reason. If they are digested slowly, there is a greater chance of undigested residues reaching the bacteria lower in the gut!

Nevertheless, it is sensible for patients with anxiety and air swallowing to have a snack – choosing low-GI foods – between breakfast and lunch, and again during the afternoon, to reduce the possibility of problems with a fall in blood sugar. If you are intolerant of wheat and cheese, a chicken drumstick or a hard-boiled egg will provide an excellent alternative. Avoid refined sugars such as sucrose jam and sweets at all cost!

OTHER CAUSES OF AIR SWALLOWING

Acid reflux causes stomach acid to flow back from the stomach into the lower gullet, causing heartburn. Many sufferers unconsciously swallow saliva to neutralise the acid and to relieve the pain. But each swallow may carry only a small amount of saliva down into the gullet. In its place, air is swallowed and collects in the stomach. A blocked nose, for example due to injury, allergy (such as hay fever), or inflammation, is a common cause of air swallowing because it forces us to breathe through the mouth. A proportion of the air we breathe into our mouths tends to go down into the stomach.

ACID REFLUX

Acid should be treated promptly with medication that reduces the acid secreted by the stomach. There will then be less acid to reflux back into the lower gullet and less heartburn. There will then be less need to swallow saliva – and air with it. Losing weight and giving up smoking can also help. Certain foods may make reflux worse such as orange juice, strong coffee, red wine and fatty meals. Try to avoid too much bending, straining to pass stools and urine or wearing tight clothing, all of which may increase the pressure inside your abdomen. Your doctor may prescribe treatment to reduce the production of acid in the stomach.

If acid reflux at night in bed is a problem, it sometimes helps to raise the head of the bed by a few inches by putting something under the legs such as a brick or books. If, despite these measures, heartburn persists, it may be due to hiatus hernia, where part of the stomach gets trapped in the gap in the diaphragm where the oesophagus passes through. This can often be treated by keyhole surgery.

BLOCKED NOSE

Hay fever can cause a blocked nose. It may only occur at certain times of the year, but some people have chronic rhinitis that is present all the year round. Treatment with nasal drops and sprays containing corticosteroids may reduce the swelling of the lining of the nose and allow air to pass through unobstructed. Allergy to house dust mite is sometimes a cause of chronic rhinitis, and your GP can advise you on how best to reduce your exposure to this.

Chronic rhinitis is sometimes caused by food intolerance. In the first instance you should try to cut out all dairy products as they are the commonest group of foods to cause this particular problem. If dairy products aren't the answer and rhinitis is chronic and severe, it may be worthwhile trying a full exclusion diet (see Chapter 5). A broken nose can cause the internal nasal passages to become completely blocked and may require surgery. If simple drops and sprays don't clear your nasal passages successfully, ask your doctor whether it would be worthwhile going to see an ENT surgeon.

Hypnosis for IBS

When treatment for IBS has been so unsatisfactory for so long, it is not surprising that many different approaches have been tried. In 1984, Professor Peter Whorwell from Manchester reported excellent results when severe IBS was treated by hypnotherapy. Thirty patients who had failed to respond to conventional therapy were put into two groups, one of which received a course of hypnotherapy. After three months that group was very much improved compared to the others with respect to all the symptoms recorded.

Since then a number of further studies have been done, and it is now generally agreed that hypnotherapy has a substantial effect on IBS. As many as 87 per cent may experience benefit, with bowel symptoms expected to improve by about half. Psychological symptoms and life functioning also improve. Furthermore, these improvements are maintained; in one group of 204 patients, 71 per cent improved initially, and only 19 per cent reported deteriorating during the following five years.

The major difficulties with hypnotherapy are that it takes time, is expensive and in Britain is not generally available on the NHS. These factors inevitably limit its use. I believe that hypnotherapy should therefore be reserved for those cases for which it is most suitable. These are not those with malfermentation or constipation, for hypnotherapy only offers relief of bowel

---

symptoms in around half these cases, much less than we expect for exclusion diets or laxative regimes.

Hypnotherapy comes into its own when IBS is caused by anxiety and air swallowing. These cases form no more than 20 per cent of routine referrals to the IBS clinic in Cambridge, but at a recent meeting one of Professor Whorwell's team told me that they comprise 80 per cent of the cases seen in his clinic. Indeed, he often screens out cases of malfermentation by suggesting a low-fibre gluten-free diet for those waiting to start treatment – three months later they are so much better that hypnotherapy is no longer required. Hypnotherapy is particularly valuable for patients with phobias – be they agoraphobia (fear of the wide open spaces) or arachnophobia (fear of spiders). Dr Claude Lum used to hypnotise his patients to desensitise them from such phobias – with considerable success.

One small downside of the use of hypnotherapy in IBS is that it may lead to simplistic deductions that if a condition can be relieved by hypnotism it must be psychological and not a genuine disease. This is simply untrue. After all, hypnotherapy will relieve the pains of childbirth, and there is nothing psychological about those. If you suffer the anxiety and air-swallowing form of IBS, and have access to a good hypnotherapist, seize the opportunity!

ANXIETY

Anxiety is the feeling we get when our body responds to frightening, threatening or stressful experiences. It is called the 'flight or fight' response as the body prepares to literally run or fight. The most common responses are:

➤ Heart beats faster.

➤ Muscles tense.

➤ Faster breathing.

➤ Sweating.

➤ Desire to go to the toilet.

Many of the stresses we face today can't be fought against or run away from, so the symptoms don't help, especially if they are not understood. Anxiety at some levels can be helpful, for example, when we need to perform well or cope in an emergency, but long-term anxiety is not helpful because:

➤ Symptoms of anxiety, while NOT dangerous, can be uncomfortable.

➤ Symptoms can be frightening to someone not used to the feelings.

➤ Sometimes people with anxiety symptoms worry they might have something seriously wrong with them. This worry can then produce more anxiety symptoms which increase the worry – and so a vicious circle is established.

➤ It can become a problem when the symptoms are severe, go on too long, happen too often, cause constant worry that there is a serious problem, or stop you doing what you want to do.

➤ It often becomes entrenched as the brain learns the pattern and the thoughts and behaviour keep the anxiety going.

CAUSES OF ANXIETY

Anxiety can affect people in the way they think, feel, and behave and how their body works. There may be many reasons why someone becomes anxious:

➤ Some people have anxious personalities and have learnt to worry.

➤ Others have a series of stressful life events to cope with, e.g. death, divorce, redundancy, house moving.

➤ Others may have pressure at work or home.

HOW TO MANAGE YOUR ANXIETY

You can learn ways of reducing anxiety and managing it. The four areas to tackle are:

➤ Understanding what makes you anxious.

➤ Reducing the physical symptoms.

➤ Changing your thought processes.

➤ Changing your behaviour.

It may help to keep a diary for at least two weeks. Rate your anxiety from 0–10 and note down all the details of any situations in which you felt anxious, and who was with you, where you were, what was your fear and so on. This will help you to identify the triggers that cause anxiety to build up. Once these have been identified you can work on solving them. Write down as many possible solutions as you can and don't be afraid to ask your GP for help. Apart from resolving the underlying problems, relaxation techniques are the only cure for anxiety. Once you can recognise the early signs of anxiety, you can reduce the severity and, in some cases, remove the anxiety and physical symptoms.

RELAXATION EXERCISES

Relaxation is important, not only to treat abnormal breathing but also to relieve anxiety and stress. Try to do the exercises once a day and as you get better at them, try to use the techniques in stressful situations. Find a comfortable position with every part of your body fully supported. If you are lying flat on the bed, put a pillow under your knees. Keep warm and choose a time you will not be disturbed.

1. Make yourself comfortable and close your eyes. Concentrate first on your feet and toes. Just let your toes feel nice and loose and let your feet feel very heavy, like lead weights at the end of your legs. They may feel so heavy that they begin to sink into the bed.

2. Think about your calf muscles and feel any tension or tightness draining away so that, from being tight and tense, they become limp and floppy and relaxed. Your lower legs now feel heavy and begin to sink into the bed like your feet.

3. Concentrate on the muscles in your thighs, at the back and the front. Release any tension there may be in them so your thigh muscles become limp, floppy and relaxed. Now both legs from top to bottom feel very heavy indeed and sink deeper and deeper into the bed the more you relax them.

4. Check the muscles in your seat. Make sure they are not squeezed together and feel loose and relaxed. Try to get the feeling of giving your weight up to the bed. Let the bed take your weight. Let it do all the work for you. From the waist down, all you have to think about doing is sinking into the bed deeper and deeper the more you relax.

5. Now think about the muscles in your back, all the way along your spine on each side. Again just feel the tension of the day draining away as you let your back muscles go. Now your back muscles are nice and relaxed and your trunk is sinking down into the bed so that the upper half of your body begins to feel as heavy and relaxed as the lower half.

6. Think about your hands and fingers. Just let your fingers rest quite loosely on the bed and let your hands feel very heavy, very limp and very floppy, so floppy that if someone was to pick up your hand and drop it, they would see it flop back like a dead weight. And as you get better at relaxing you may loose the feeling in your fingers. This is quite normal when you relax deeply.

7. Think about the muscles in your forearms. Just feel tension flowing away so that your forearms, too, become heavy and sink into the bed along with the rest of you. Do the same with the muscles in the top half of your arms. Let them go. Let them relax so that both arms from top to bottom feel very heavy indeed and may even feel as if they do not belong to you at all.

8. Next we come to the muscles around your shoulders, especially across the back of your shoulders. As you try to relax them, almost feel your shoulders dropping just that little bit further still so that they feel very low, very saggy and very relaxed.

9. Let your head fall back into the pillow wherever it wants to. Let the pillow take the weight of your head so that your neck muscles can also relax. Think of it as a large triangular area down the

back of your neck to the tips of both shoulders, a triangle very prone to tension. Loosen as much of that tension as you can by letting your shoulders down and your head fall heavily into the pillow.

10. Check the muscles across the top part of your chest. Loosen any tight feeling you have across your upper chest so that your chest is as still as possible and you are letting the air down to your diaphragm so gently and easily that the air almost bypasses that top part of your chest.

11. Let your tongue fall loosely in your mouth. Let the muscles go at the angles of your jaw so that your lower jaw feels loose and heavy. Let the muscles go across your forehead so that you do not feel that you are frowning and let them go around your eyes so that your eyes are just gently closed. Your whole face now should be totally relaxed and free from any expression whatsoever.

12. Now think about relaxing your body as a whole unit from head to foot. Think about breathing slowly and gently from your diaphragm. Each time you breathe out, it is like releasing any tension that you have left along with the air you expel. Each time you breathe out, aim to feel a little bit heavier still. Each time you breathe out, sink a little bit deeper into the bed. The only effort you have to make is when you breathe in. When you breathe out let everything go. You are letting go of the air, letting go of tension with that air and letting go of yourself. As you breathe out just relax.

13. Now try to relax mentally. Imagine you are standing at the top of a flight of 10 steps. Picture

yourself going down the steps one by one, relaxing with each step that you take. See yourself take the first step, relaxing as you go. Then the second, third, fourth, fifth, sixth, seventh, eighth, ninth and now the last.

14. Picture yourself sitting or lying in whichever place you choose, somewhere very lovely, very peaceful and very calm and picture that place all around you as clearly as you can. Not only seeing it around you but maybe hearing the things that may be going on there and just feeling the atmosphere of peace and quiet. While you are thinking about that place, go on breathing gently and slowly with your diaphragm and go on relaxing each time you breathe out.

15. Stay here relaxing, breathing slowly and visualising your beautiful place for as long as you wish. When you are ready to finish, climb up the stairs in your mind, open your eyes at the top and when you feel ready you can get up and go about your daily routine.

OTHER RELAXATION METHODS

In addition to this exercise, find your own preference for relaxation. It may be a yoga class or self- hypnosis tape. A relaxation CD or audio tape, ideally with headphones, has also been of benefit to patients. You might find it useful to read the above technique out loud and record it so that you can play it back to yourself, following the instructions. Alternatively, you can purchase one at www.ibsessentials.co.uk (see Further Information, page 195.)

We find that 80 per cent of our patients gain considerable relief from symptoms by following the set exercises, and learning to relax and breathe correctly with the diaphragm. Although all the above exercises may appear rather daunting, the results we have seen have been excellent in those patients who have stuck to the exercises.

In a Papworth study by Dr Lum of patients with anxiety treated with the exercise regime described in this chapter, out of 320 cases, 70 per cent were completely symptom free after one year, 25 per cent had only minor symptoms and 5 per cent failed to respond. More recently, this success rate tallies with our personal experience of patients in our clinic. The message is that if you can do the exercises regularly and for a good period of time, then enormous progress can be made in the eradication of symptoms of air swallowing.

Emotional Freedom Technique (EFT)

This is an alternative way of dealing with anxiety and this could help with the symptoms of IBS. EFT is a form of emotional acupuncture that does not use needles and that you can easily learn to do on yourself. It is a new class of treatment in the field of energy psychology. It was founded by Gary Craig, a Stanford engineer who based his work on Einstein's theory that all things (including our bodies) are made of energy. By tapping with your fingers on certain specific acupuncture points on the body's energy meridians (mainly head and hands), you can release blocks in your energy system that may be contributing to your symptoms of IBS. You can download the training manual for EFT at www.emofree.com or find a practitioner in your area to get you started – they are all listed on the website as well.

Several clients of mine have reported significant improvement in dealing not only with the anxiety that accompanies IBS, but also with the symptoms them-selves. Another recommended method of training yourself how to cope with anxiety is the Linden Method (www.thelindenmethod.co.uk). Here we see how Charles Linden cured himself of panic and anxiety attacks and he has devised a method that is recognised by GPs.

SUMMARY

➤ Some IBS symptoms, especially pain due to bloating and excess wind, may be due to air swallowing and/or anxiety.

➤ Air swallowing can be due to abnormal breathing patterns — breathing too rapidly and too shallowly — among other causes, especially when you are anxious or excited.

➤ Exercises to improve your breathing can have a dramatic effect on symptoms in many cases — see page 100.

➤ Anxiety not only increases the likelihood of air swallowing but may worsen IBS symptoms in its own right.

➤ Identifying underlying causes of anxiety and using relaxation techniques (see page 113) can help.

➤ Hypnotherapy has also been effective in tackling the underlying psychological causes of anxiety that can cause IBS symptoms.

CHAPTER 8

CONSTIPATION

Some people are confused about the distinction between simple constipation and IBS. In a nutshell, the difference hinges on whether or not there is any *abdominal pain*. Because the committees in Rome drew up separate criteria for both IBS and for constipation, it would be easy to believe that this meant that the two were quite different conditions. This is not so. The essential difference is that IBS produces abdominal pain, but that constipation may not. Many people who are constipated have little, if any, pain, and thus do not fit the Rome criteria for IBS. The following advice is equally relevant to constipation, whether it is associated with pain or not.

Constipation is a vitally important cause of IBS. It is crucial to recognise it, in all its various forms, for if it is not corrected, then the IBS it produces will not be treated successfully. A normal bowel habit may be quite variable. The frequency of 'normal' bowel movements may vary from three times a day to three times a week! However, a definition of constipation that depends simply on the number of times you empty your bowels no longer suffices to cover all the difficulties that may arise.

The time taken for food waste to pass out of the body – the whole gut transit time (WGTT: see page 25) – may be prolonged in people who pass a stool every day. The bowels are open, but the large intestine is not emptied adequately. So it's now customary to include further problems in the definition of constipation. The other most common feature of constipation is that the faeces are hard and difficult to pass. Constipation is the underlying reason for many cases of IBS. In order to treat this type of IBS successfully, it is necessary to understand the causes of the constipation, and to relieve it.

At the same time that the group of doctors meeting in Rome were drawing up the Rome II Criteria for diagnosing IBS they were also drafting a definition of constipation (below). As you can see, it's quite complex.

ROME II CRITERIA FOR CONSTIPATION

Adults

Two or more of the following symptoms for at least 12 weeks or more (not necessarily consecutive), in the preceding 12 months:

1. Straining in more than 25 per cent of bowel movements.

2. Lumpy or hard stools for more than 25 per cent of bowel movements.

3. Sensation of incomplete emptying of the bowel for more than 25 per cent of bowel movements.

4. Sensation of blockage in the anus and lower rectum for more than 25 per cent of bowel movements.

5. A need to use the hand to help the bowel emptying in more than 25 per cent of occasions. This could include pressure to help the bowel to empty or digital evacuation.

6. Less than three bowel movements per week.

Infants and Children

1. Pebble-like or hard stools for the majority of bowel movements for at least two weeks.

2. Firm stools more than twice a week for at least two weeks.

3. No evidence of structural abnormalities or other disease.

THE NORMAL BEHAVIOUR OF THE LARGE INTESTINE

The digestion of food and absorption of nutrients mainly occurs in the small intestine. Waste residues then pass into the large intestine, or bowel, where they are fermented by billions of helpful bacteria, producing nutrients such as vitamins and fatty acids. Toxic chemicals are broken down and water absorbed back into the body. Mucus is secreted by the large bowel to bind the contents together and to protect the gut wall as the residue is compacted into a semi-solid mass. Faeces are made up of bacteria, water, protein, fat, undigested roughage and dead cells shed from the lining of the bowel.

Normal defecation involves a co-ordinated contraction of the diaphragm and the muscles of the abdominal wall. This, together with contractions of muscles in the wall of the bowel, known as peristalsis, pushes the faeces along the bowel and into the rectum. Its presence here triggers the urge to empty the bowel. This involves a complex reflex that sends information to the spinal cord and back again to trigger the muscles into expelling the stool. This reflex is involuntary, but we can override it. The muscles of the pelvic floor and the sphincter in the anus act as stoppers for the lower bowel, preventing us from passing faeces until we are ready. I call this combination of muscles 'the cork'. We can consciously prevent them from relaxing and so control the urge to defecate. Relaxing the muscles of the pelvic floor and the anal sphincters straightens out the angle between the rectum and the anus and allows faeces to pass through.

In some people, constipation is associated with a failure to relax the muscles that narrow the angle between the anus and the rectum or even inappropriately to contract them. This increases the pressure in the anal canal itself so that the stool is not able to pass through easily.

Eating food stretches the stomach and this triggers peristalsis in the large bowel, a reflex known as the gastro-colic reflex. This reflex is usually suppressed until we are ready to go to the lavatory because we have positive control over our bowel actions. Bowel activity also varies during the day. On waking it increases and this is why many people need to visit the lavatory first thing in the morning. Bowel activity slows in the afternoon, particularly if people are inactive or having a nap.

When you are asleep at night, the colon slows almost to a standstill. This encourages fermentation to proceed and this is why more colonic gas is produced while we sleep. Bowel activity is increased by exercise. The combination of this and the gastro-colic reflex means that those who are physically active often need to visit the lavatory after a meal. Finally, bowel movement is affected by psychological factors. It takes longer for the contents to pass through the large bowel in people who are distressed, for example.

CAUSES OF CONSTIPATION

Causes of constipation fall into six main groups:

POOR BOWEL HABITS

Faulty technique when going to the lavatory is a common cause of constipation. For example, straining is a frequent fault that may cause lots of difficulties with opening your bowels as it can lead to incorrect action of the pelvic floor muscles. If these do not hold the anus in position, increases in abdominal pressure may just force the anus downwards, when it becomes hard to push the faeces through it. If they do not relax to straighten the rectum and open the anus, the stools cannot pass through at all. Signs of straining include:

➤ Gulping in a breath of air before trying to defecate.

➤ Keeping the lips tightly closed.

➤ Sucking in the stomach muscles rather than letting them bulge forward.

➤ Supporting the stomach muscles with your hands when trying to pass a stool.

➤ Trying to push down into the toilet bowl.

Many women develop faulty bowel habits because they do not sit in the right position on the loo. When we are small children, standard adult lavatories are too big for us. Children are scared that they may fall right down inside, and so perch on the edge of the seat. As we grow, boys are forced to sit back, for if they don't and they pass urine, it goes all over the floor. Girls, on the other hand, often continue to perch on the edge of the seat into adult life. Busy, multi-tasking women may begrudge time spent in the lavatory, and the combination of haste and a poor position can lead to real problems with opening the bowel. For advice on how to sit in the correct position on the loo, see pages 131–132.

DIET AND LIFESTYLE

The amount of faeces present and its consistency are important factors in the speed at which it passes though the gut. Fluid intake is clearly important. If we don't drink enough, the motions may become hard and difficult to pass. Ideally we should all drink two to three litres of water a day – more if the weather is hot or we are exercising vigorously. Increasing fibre in the diet may help not only to prevent constipation, but also diverticular disease, piles and faecal incontinence. A lack of fibre, dehydration, rushed lifestyle and travel may all affect the consistency of the stools and lead to constipation.

SLUGGISH BOWEL

If the bowel muscles don't contract properly, its contents will not progress. This may occur to a mild extent in people without any specific bowel disease. Women who are pregnant frequently develop constipation and many women also notice mild problems just before their periods. Sometimes the passage of faeces along the bowel may become sluggish (slow transit constipation) for no obvious reason at all. The muscle of the gut may be damaged by diseases such as scleroderma and slowed by certain drugs, particularly painkillers containing codeine, or by iron tablets, used to treat anaemia.

WEAKENED PELVIC FLOOR

The muscles of the pelvic floor, which support the organs of the lower abdomen, are important in preventing incontinence over long periods. During defecation it is essential that they relax to allow the stool to pass easily through. If the pelvic floor muscles are weakened, for example during pregnancy and childbirth, there can be an involuntary release of urine or faeces, especially when coughing or lifting. You can strengthen them by doing pelvic floor exercises (see below).

UNDERLYING DISEASE

A number of conditions affecting the brain and the nervous system will affect the large bowel, including stress, depression dementia, disease of the spinal cord, or conditions such as multiple sclerosis. Damage to nerves supplying the gut, for example following childbirth or hysterectomy, is another important factor. Anything that affects the urge to open the bowels may lead to constipation. This includes local painful conditions such as fissures in the anus, haemorrhoids, or abnormalities of its nerves as in Hirschsprung's disease, or by damage to the nerves supplying the rectum which leads to reduced sensation there. The lining of the rectum may be forced downwards when the bowel contracts. Such pressures may hinder the passage of the faeces or may be severe enough to lead to ulcers in the rectum and even, on occasion, prolapse of the rectum, which causes it to protrude out through the anus.

The bowel can become narrowed as a result of tumours, Crohn's disease or diverticulitis and this may obstruct the passage of faeces. Pressure on the bowel from outside may arise from adhesions, which are bands of scar tissue following previous surgery or infection.

MEDICATION

Many drugs can cause gastrointestinal disturbances, including painkillers, antacids and iron supplements (see below), but any drug may potentially have this effect. If your constipation comes on after a change in treatment, you must always discuss it with your doctor.

DRUGS THAT CAUSE CONSTIPATION

Painkillers: opiates	Codeine, Coproxamol
Non-steroidal anti-inflammatory agents (NSAIDs)	Aspirin, Nurofen
Drugs affecting peristalsis: Anti-spasmodics	Buscopan, Merbeverine
Anti-depressants	Amitriptyline
Anti-psychotics	
Some drugs used in the treatment of Parkinson's disease	
Drugs containing metals: Iron supplements	
Aluminium (antacids)	Antacids
Other agents Anti-hypertensive drugs (for high blood pressure)	
Anti-convulsants (for epilepsy) Cholesterol-reducing drugs	Simvastatin

TREATMENT OF CONSTIPATION

The long list of possible causes of constipation shows that it is not a disease in its own right, but a symptom that may arise for many different reasons. If constipation develops, it is essential that you first see your GP to make sure there is no serious cause underlying it, such as a tumour or a stricture in the bowel. Before following the suggestions given here, see your doctor to ensure more serious causes have been excluded. It's always a mistake to attempt self-diagnosis.

LIFESTYLE CHANGES

Consider changes in lifestyle that may help your bowel to function more efficiently. Try to develop a regular bowel habit by taking time to go to the lavatory at the same time each day. Many people find it's convenient after breakfast, when bowel activity is increasing and when the added stimulus of eating a meal is present. However, if you prefer to go at another time of day, choose that time and stick to it.

1. **Exercise** can increase bowel activity. The physical activity does not need to be particularly vigorous. A session at the gym can help, but many people find it's enough to take a regular walk, maybe with the dog, or doing gardening or even housework. Swimming and cycling are other possibilities.

2. **Don't put off going to the lavatory**. When you feel the urge, make time to go. Repeated suppression of the urge, for example because you are busy, causes the nerves in the rectum to become less sensitive so that the normal reflexes are dulled and constipation may get worse.

3. **Improve your diet**. Drink plenty of fluid (2–3 litres) throughout the day – especially water. It's important to have plenty of fibre in your diet, too, but be careful which sort you choose. Those who have constipation

with excess wind need to obtain sufficient residue to keep their bowels busy while also reducing fermentation in order to cut down the amount of wind they produce. Non-fermentable bulk-forming fibre (such as linseed) is usually best as its passes through the bowel, drawing in fluid and increasing the bulk of the stools without being broken down itself and producing extra gas and bloating. At the same time you should reduce the fermentable fibre in your diet. Wheat bran, for example, leads to excess gas production, bloating and pain.

We shall discuss later whether it is sensible to try an exclusion diet in the management of constipation. In the first instance, however, the diet below provides a sensible approach.

UNDERSTANDING FIBRE

Dietary fibre includes those substances that resist digestion in the small intestine and pass into the large bowel where the process of fermentation begins. It broadly incorporates three categories:

1. Resistant starch.

2. Soluble fibre.

3. Insoluble fibre.

Other compounds such as complex sugars may ultimately be found to be important, particularly in their role as prebiotics (See Chapter 9). Fibre can be subdivided according to its ability to absorb water. Soluble fibre such as pectin, guar or ispaghula takes up water to form a jelly-like solution that is easily acceptable to bacterial enzymes and rapidly fermented to produce gases such as hydrogen and methane and other important chemicals such as short-chain fatty acids. Soluble fibre is found in oats, pulses (peas, beans and lentils) and most fruit and vegetables. In general, little or no soluble fibre is recoverable from faeces.

Insoluble fibre such as cellulose can bind water but does not form a solution and so is more resistant to fermentation. It tends to be excreted in larger amounts and thus may have a greater laxative effect. The substances in these categories include all the bulking agents (see page 91) such as sterculia and methyl cellulose.

While about 10–20 g of insoluble fibre reaches the large bowel daily in the normal diet, the remainder of 'dietary fibre' comes in the form of resistant starch. Starch is a complex chemical made up of chains of sugars and the majority of it is easily digested in the small intestine by enzymes released by the pancreas. However, some starch reaches the large bowel and is fermented.

Cooking may alter resistant starch so that it can be digested, by altering its structure, but the structure may reform when the food cools. Thus freshly cooked potato and rice are generally easily digested and absorbed, but cold potato and cold rice contain resistant starch that may cause excess fermentation, wind and bloating.

Even more important than whether fibre is soluble or insoluble is its resistance to fermentation. Thus, although all forms of fibre will increase the speed of passage of food through the gut, and make stools softer and bulkier, in IBS patients it can lead to over-production of wind, causing pain and bloating. Fibre supplements used in IBS, therefore, should ideally be poorly fermented. Sterculia, linseed and methyl cellulose are the most easily available.

HIGH-FIBRE DIET

A high-fibre diet suitable for constipation includes the following:

➤ Wholemeal, granary and soft-grain varieties of bread.

➤ Jacket potatoes, new potatoes in their skins and baked potato skins.

➤ Wholegrain breakfast cereals, e.g. Weetabix, bran flakes, unsweetened muesli, Shreddies and porridge oats.

➤ Wholemeal pasta and brown rice.

➤ Beans, lentils and peas.

➤ Fresh and dried fruits – particularly if the skins are eaten.

➤ Vegetables – particularly if the skins are eaten (lettuce, tomatoes, potatoes peeled or mashed, pumpkin, cucumber, courgettes, marrow, green beans, lentils, peas, leeks, shallots, celery, parsley, garlic, asparagus, beetroot, turnip, swede).

➤ Nuts and seeds.

➤ Wholemeal flour.

Dietary fibre should be increased gradually by including one or two new high-fibre foods each week. Rather than simply adding bran to foods, try adding a variety of fruit and vegetable sources (from the above list). For example, have salad every day as a meal or side order, plus a daily fruit salad. Include different starchy foods, including bread, pita bread and rice. This ensures a good mixture of soluble fibre (found mainly in fruits and vegetables, pulses and oats) and insoluble fibre (found mainly in cereal products), each of which has different beneficial effects on bowel function. It is important that you increase fluid intake at the same time as increasing fibre.

A high-fibre diet should be tried for about four weeks to see if it is helpful. If the constipation is not resolved, or if the high-fibre diet is not well-tolerated, laxatives – especially bulking agents — may be tried instead (see below).

COMPARISON OF BULKING AGENTS AND FERMENTATION

BULKING AGENT	ACTIVE COMPONENT	FIBRE TYPE	FERMENTATION
Wheat bran	wheat bran	insoluble	Slow and incomplete
Celevac	methyl cellulose	insoluble	Variable resistance depending on the size of the molecules
Fybogel, Regulan, Isogel	ispaghula husk	soluble	Moderate; 20–30% excreted
Normacol	sterculia	soluble	Resistant
Linseeds	linseed husk	insoluble	Resistant

GOING TO THE LOO PROPERLY

The natural position for humans to pass a motion is squatting. The introduction of the lavatory subtly changed this so it is essential that you sit back comfortably on the seat, leaning slightly forward, shoulders, arms and legs relaxed. If possible, sit on the toilet with your knees slightly higher than your hips (it may help to use a small stool or books to raise your feet). The abdominal wall is then pushed out, increasing the pressure inside and also encouraging the anus to reflex and the muscles of the pelvic floor to relax. Keep the back straight, flexing forwards slightly from the hips; the diaphragm then moves down pressing the abdominal contents against the rectum. A series of well-timed pushes empties the left side of the bowel.

EXERCISES TO IMPROVE YOUR PERFORMANCE

The key first step is to allow the muscles of the abdominal wall to bulge forward, thus increasing abdominal pressure. It may be a helpful exercise to train the 'six pack' muscle at the front of the abdomen (*rectus abdominis*). Push it out for 10 seconds – this is called making it 'bold'. You will notice your breathing stops as your diaphragm moves down. Practise this technique every day four to six times for one to two minutes.

If despite this you still have difficulties, you may brace the abdominal muscles by putting your hands over your lower ribs just above your waist. Push your abdominal muscles out to the side and hold. This has the effect of making your waist wider and is called bracing. If you 'bold' your abdominal wall and brace the muscles in this way three to four times quickly, you may find you can move the faeces further down into the lower rectum. Sustain the action as you feel the faeces going through your anus.

This exercise is also helpful when you think you have finished to see if you really are empty. If you brace and bold several times, it will evacuate any faeces that may be left. If nothing else comes, you have really finished and if there is a temptation to go back to your old straining habits, don't! If the urge remains strong, go and lie down for a few minutes and it will pass.

PELVIC FLOOR EXERCISES

To find your pelvic floor, pretend you are trying to stop yourself urinating or passing wind. When you do this, you will feel a tightening around your bladder, rectum and vagina/testicles. This is your pelvic floor. By tightening your pelvic floor on a regular basis you strengthen the muscles and so help improve bowel function. Try to do the following exercises several times a day. You can do them anywhere, in the car, on a train, waiting for the kettle to boil, as no one can see you do them.

1. Breathing normally, contract and then immediately relax your pelvic floor. Do this up to five times. As your muscles get stronger, over the days and weeks, increase the number of quick contractions you do up to a maximum of 10 times.

2. Breathing normally, contract your pelvic floor and hold for a count of five, and then relax. Do this up to five times. As your muscles get stronger, over the days and weeks, increase the length of time you contract your pelvic floor up to a maximum of 10 seconds.

IF LIFESTYLE CHANGES DON'T WORK

If you've tried the life-style suggestions and corrected any deficiencies there and still your problems persist, follow the guidance given regarding overload and overflow (page 88) to empty the bowel completely using a bowel cleansing agent such as Picolax or Citramag. Purges of this sort are not meant to be used as treatments for constipation. They are too strong to be taken regularly, and should be used only as an occasional way of emptying the bowel. They should be followed by use of non-fementable bulk-forming agents in order to allow milder forms of laxative to work effectively. Other forms of laxative may be helpful, too, such as osmotic agents and stimulants. The following are the main laxatives commonly used.

LAXATIVES

The use of laxatives goes back to the very beginnings of our civilisation. Many were derived from herbs and plants, but that doesn't necessarily mean that they were mild and harmless. Some – such as aloes, colocynth and jalap – have effects that are too powerful and may deplete the body of water and essential salts, such as potassium. Therefore, as a general rule, the mildest possible laxative should be used.

Bulk-forming agents

Also known as bulking agents, these are very popular because they work by re-enforcing the natural physiology of the bowel. They relieve constipation by increasing the residue in the stool, which draws fluid into it thereby increasing its mass and which, in turn, stimulates peristalsis. This results in a larger, soft and easily-passed stool. It is therefore very important that they are taken together with plenty of fluid.

They are of particular value in those people who pass small, hard stools. They are in general fairly mild, and it is thus important that they are started after the bowel has been cleared, for by themselves they are not strong enough to clear out the colon. Giving a bulk-forming agent to someone with a loaded colon will just make their bloating worse.

➤ Sterculia and linseed: These are the best ones to use as they are least likely to cause bloating and flatulence. Some bulk-forming laxatives are fermented by colonic bacteria, which may cause uncomfortable wind and distension in those with IBS and should be avoided (see also page 91).

Osmotic agents

These are effective because they are not absorbed, but are retained within the gut. They therefore draw fluid into the bowel, making the stools larger and softer. Osmotic agents include magnesium salts, unabsorbable sugars such as lactulose, and polyethylene glycol.

➤ Magnesium salts: Magnesium sulphate (Epsom salts) and magnesium hydroxide mixture (Milk of Magnesia) are all effective laxatives. Magnesium salts are not suitable for people with kidney disease as the level of magnesium in the blood may rise too high. Milpar is magnesium hydroxide combined with liquid paraffin and also acts as a stool softener (se below).

➤ Lactulose: This is a sugar that cannot be digested in the gut and therefore passes all the way down the bowel, drawing in fluid as it goes. As it is a sugar, it is fermented by bacteria when it reaches the large bowel and can then give rise to wind, bloating and discomfort. Some microbiologists claim that this is an advantage, as lactulose then acts as a prebiotic (see Chapter 9) and may promote the growth of healthy *Bifidobacteria* and *Lactobacilli*. However, to my mind the practical difficulties of wind and pain outweigh this theoretical gain, and I therefore rarely recommend it for use in IBS.

➤ *Polyethylene glycol* (Macrogols): This inert chemical passes right through the bowel without being broken down in any way. It keeps fluid in the bowel and so has less of a dehydrating effect than some of the other osmotic laxatives.

Stimulants

These act on the muscles in the wall of the bowel causing them to contract, thus promoting peristalsis and faecal expulsion. A lot of them are herbal or natural laxatives. Some such as aloes, colocynth and jalap should be avoided as they have a drastic purgative action. Other natural laxatives such as cascara, frangula, rhubarb and senna-pods may vary in strength because of their natural origin. This means their action is unpredictable and so they, too, should be avoided.

All stimulant laxatives increase bowel movement and so may cause abdominal cramps. There is still anxiety about the prolonged use of these laxatives as the dose required tends to increase with time, and as it is claimed that they can precipitate weakness of the gut muscles leading to a feeble non-contracting large bowel. But it is quite harmless to take them on an occasional basis, and I often suggest that patients use them once or twice a week.

➤ Senna: This is particularly valuable as the total amount of senna contained is standardised, so that its laxative effect is predictable.

➤ *Sodium picosulphate*: This is the active component of Picolax, which is too powerful for use other than as a bowel-cleansing solution. But sodium picosulphate is also available in a much lower dose as an elixir or as Dulco-lax Perles and is often useful in stubborn cases. **Laxatives that contain a lot of sodium may be inadvisable for patients with high blood pressure and heart disease,** so see your doctor first.

➤ Glycerine suppositories: These contain glycerol, which is mildly irritant.

How to Use a Suppository

Suppositories have to be inserted deep into the rectum past the anal sphincters. To do this properly, squat and push out the front of your belly to open the anus. Put in the suppository from the front of your body as this enables it to run along the posterior wall of the bowel into a higher satisfactory position.

Stool softeners

Liquid paraffin (which is also a constituent of Milpar – see above) was once widely used but is now less popular because there is a risk of paraffin getting into the lungs causing damage (lipoid pneumonia). Docusate Sodium (Dulco-ease) is a softening agent that may also have a stimulant effect.

Which laxative should I use?

It is sensible to discuss with your doctor which laxatives are likely to be best for you. In general, however, the principle is to empty the bowel completely and to follow up, using the smallest effective dose possible, with a harmless laxative. Bulk laxatives are the most simple and straightforward to use. Sterculia and linseed are the ones least likely to cause bloating and flatulence.

If bulking agents alone are insufficient, I usually suggest adding an osmotic agent – perhaps a magnesium salt. Polyethylene glycol (Movicol) is particularly useful in the elderly. If you are still having problems, then the best combination is likely to be a bulking agent supplemented by occasional doses of a stimulant laxative, such as Senokot, Bisacodyl or sodium picosulphate elixir.

WHAT ABOUT AN EXCLUSION DIET?

We have had a number of patients who have been able to control their constipation very successfully by means of food exclusion. However, I would only suggest trying an exclusion diet when laxatives and a low-fibre diet have not been successful in controlling the constipation and the pain of IBS satisfactorily. If you also suffer other symptoms that are commonly produced by food intolerance, such as a stuffy nose, headaches, fluid retention and tiredness, the chances of success are improved.

If you do decide to try an exclusion diet, take a non-fermentable laxative such as sterculia at the same time and continue on the basic diet for two to three weeks only. If, at the end of this time, the bowel function is not clearly satisfactory with three or more motions each week and a considerable reduction in abdominal pain, then stop the diet and ask your GP about other ways forward.

If the stool frequency and the pain do improve, then the process of food testing must be carried out very carefully. Read the advice and suggestions given in Chapter 5 and test each food over a much longer period than is usually allowed. I suggest a minimum of four to five days for each food. This is clearly going to be a slow and tedious business, but if the constipation is satisfactorily resolved on the basic diet, it will be worthwhile.

WHAT IF I AM STILL HAVING PROBLEMS WITH MY BOWELS?

If you initially thought that your problem was slow-transit constipation, but the advice you have read here has not done the trick – then think again. Could it be that you have obstructed defecation all the time? Why not read on, and see how you progress.

YOU WANT TO GO BUT YOU CAN'T – OBSTRUCTED DEFECATION

The control of constipation mainly depends on diet, adequate fluid intake, exercise and appropriate laxatives. Some people, however, still find they are unable to go. Indeed they may feel they want to go quite badly, but frustratingly they find that they can't.

This is called obstructed defecation and usually happens in women. There are a number of possible reasons for this. Giving birth may have caused damage to the pelvic nerves or the pelvic floor muscles which they supply. Repeated straining to empty the bowels is another reason. When you try to empty the bowel the pelvic floor can become over-stretched and the perineum (the area between the vagina/scrotum and the anus) moves down further than normal, pushing the anus so far below its usual position that the muscles that normally open it no longer work.

Other causes of obstructed defecation include prolapse of the uterus. This may allow the wall of the rectum to push forwards into the wall of the vagina, which has become slack, to form a bulge called a rectocoele. This makes passing a motion difficult because increased abdominal pressure then pushes the faeces forwards into the bulge, rather than downwards into the anal canal.

Prolapse of the rectum can also occur. This means that the rectum is pushed down towards the anus, so that parts of it may even protrude outside. Minor degrees of prolapse may affect only the lining of the rectum, which, during defecation, may be pushed down so hard that the tissue is stretched and its blood supply affected so that an ulcer forms. This causes pain and bleeding, which make matters even more difficult. Sometimes the prolapse of the rectum may be such that the rectum starts to turn in on itself or the rectal lining falls down so far as to block the anus. The rectum may even prolapse through the anus to appear outside the body.

Obstructed defecation may cause so much difficulty that patients may have to press on the skin behind the vagina or scrotum or inside the vagina to allow stools to pass at all. In severe cases they may have to remove lumps of faeces from the rectum with a finger. There may be a feeling of fullness or a lump on sitting. It's then not unusual for faeces or slime to leak onto underwear. There may be bleeding from the rectum and itchiness around the anus. Pain is common, nagging like toothache and felt in the pelvis and the lower back. There may be related effects on the bladder causing incontinence, frequency and urgency to urinate. In women there may be decreased vaginal sensation, inability to retain tampons and sex may become uncomfortable.

Sometimes these problems are so severe that surgery becomes necessary. A rectocoele may be repaired by a gynaecologist, or an operation called a rectopexy may be performed to hold up the rectal wall and stop it prolapsing. Sometimes a rectopexy may be combined with the removal of a small stretch of redundant intestine.

Surgery, however, is usually reserved for those cases that do not respond to simpler methods. It is first necessary to learn to pass stools correctly, to rehabilitate pelvic muscles and to manage pelvic pain.

BIOFEEDBACK PROGRAMME FOR CONSTIPATION

Taking control of your bowel habit may seem difficult at times, especially when you feel under stress or when the problem has continued for a long time. The following routine will help you open your bowels regularly and with ease, so that your bowel problems no longer interfere with your daily life.

Every day set aside approximately five minutes for this – ideally half an hour after breakfast. It is important that you are not interrupted. You need to push the motions downwards and you need to open the muscle in your bottom to allow the contents to pass out.

IDENTIFY THE DIFFERENT MUSCLES YOU WILL USE

1. First find your waist muscles. These are the muscles you push/propel with. Place your hands on either side of your waist. Now cough. Can you feel the muscles stiffen? When you push down you need to feel these muscles expand so that your waist becomes wider.

2. Now your anal sphincter or back passage muscle. When you go to the loo you **must** relax and open this muscle. Insert your finger just inside your back passage. Squeeze your back passage as if you were trying to stop yourself opening your bowels. It should tighten around your finger. Conversely, as you push down you should feel the muscle open and relax around your finger. Make sure that you can control this muscle and recognise when you are squeezing and when you are relaxing. Sometimes it helps to think of the muscle like a 'lift' that is on the 'ground floor'. By squeezing you can take the 'lift' up one 'floor' and by relaxing you can take the 'lift' down to the 'basement'.

CHECK YOUR SITTING POSITION ON THE TOILET

Lean forward with your forearms resting on your thighs and your feet raised. It may help to use a small stool or some books or which to rest your feet.

RELAX

Lower your shoulders. Breathe slowly and gently. In through your nose and out through your mouth. Try to let go with all your muscles and breathe so that your tummy moves up and down but not your chest (see Chapter 7 for correct breathing habits).

NOW TRY TO OPEN YOUR BOWELS

1. Sit comfortably.

2. Breathe in a relaxed way so that your muscles are not tense.

3. Close your eyes. Push down so your waist becomes wide.

4. At the same time make sure that your anal sphincter is open and relaxed.

5. Following the analogy given above, slowly push your 'lift' down to the 'basement' and hold for a few seconds and then repeat several times. You can use your brace to help you push (see below).

6. Relax for a second. Do not let the 'lift' rise back up. (Keep it in the 'basement'.)

7. Push your 'lift' down again. Repeat several times.

Remember, do NOT squeeze the muscles around your back passage but keep them relaxed, do NOT strain, and do NOT stay on the toilet for longer than 10 minutes. Remember, too, that this takes time and practice to perfect.

THE BRACE TECHNIQUE

You need to take control of your bowels. This may seem difficult at times, especially when you feel under stress. The following routine will help you to regain control. **Every day**, set aside approximately five minutes for this. (Preferably half an hour after breakfast.) It is important that you are not interrupted.

CHECK YOUR SITTING POSITION ON THE TOILET

Lean forward with your forearms resting on your thighs.

RELAX

1. Lower your shoulders.

2. Breathe slowly and gently, in through your nose and out through your mouth.

3. Try to 'let go' with all your muscles.

NOW TRY TO OPEN YOUR BOWELS

Remember **NOT** to hold your breath – do not take a big breath in first.

1. **Slowly** brace outwards (widen your waist). When fully braced, push/propel from your waist **back** and **downwards** into your back passage. **DO NOT STRAIN!**

2. Relax for one second but only slightly. You should maintain a level of pressure with your brace, while not pushing with it.

3. Brace outwards and push downwards again. This should be repeated.

You should use your brace as a pump.

Remember:

➤ This will take time and practice.

➤ Do not spend more than 10 minutes on the toilet.

➤ Do not return to the toilet unless you have a definite urge to open your bowels.

Colonic Irrigation (lavage)

There has been a vogue in recent years for colonic irrigation. Some alternative practitioners say that it not only relieves the discomfort of constipation, but it may provide all sorts of other benefits in terms of general health and energy. They maintain that sometimes the bowel becomes clogged up with faecal residues that have been present for months or longer and only a colonic washout is effective in getting rid of these. Doctors who perform endoscopic examinations of the bowel, such as sigmoidoscopy and colonoscopy, are very well aware of the best way to empty the colon. Sometimes patients are prepared for sigmoidoscopies by the nurses giving an enema. This is the equivalent of colonic lavage and only the lower part of the bowel is emptied satisfactorily in this way. When a colonoscopy is being performed, it is essential to be able to examine the entire large bowel and such enemas will not suffice. The bowel must be emptied by means of a vigorous purge, for example, using Picolax or Citramag (see page 89). Doctors therefore do not recommend colonic lavage as we know that washouts through the anus are relatively ineffective. Furthermore, passing a tube into the rectum in order to flush out the bowel carries a certain degree of risk as the colon is a delicate organ and perforations of the bowel wall which require surgery to repair them can arise in this way.

SUMMARY

➤ Constipation is a major aspect of IBS in many people and needs to be tackled.

➤ Common causes include faulty technique when going to the lavatory, lack of fibre and fluid in the diet, sluggish bowel and/or weak pelvic floor (often associated with pregnancy) and prescription drugs.

➤ In some cases, constipation may be due to underlying disease.

➤ Improved lavatory technique and lifestyle changes, such as better diet and more exercise, are the first steps to take.

➤ Strengthening the abdominal muscles – including the pelvic floor – will also help.

➤ In stubborn cases, use of a bowel cleansing agent followed by regular use of bulking agents will usually restore healthy bowel function.

CHAPTER 9

Understanding Probiotics and Prebiotics

The immune system plays a vital role in defending us against infection. One of its most important functions is to recognise and destroy invading bacteria, to which we are all exposed daily. It is not capable, however, of telling the difference between foreign bacteria that are capable of causing disease (pathogenic) and those that are quite harmless. Thus all new bacteria, be they dangerous such as *Salmonella* or possibly beneficial such as probiotic bacteria like *Lactobacilli,* are treated in the same way by the immune system and destroyed.

THE DEVELOPMENT OF A HEALTHY BACTERIAL FLORA IN THE GUT

The gut of a baby is sterile when it is born. Bacteria start to colonise the gut during the very process of birth, the baby meeting some of its mother's gut flora even as it passes down the birth canal (the gut bacteria of babies born by caesarean section are at first less complex than those born in the natural way).

Breastfeeding encourages the development of healthy gut flora. Indeed, recent research has suggests that helpful bacteria like *Lactobacilli* are absorbed from the mother's bowel and secreted in the milk itself, so that the baby gets a good supply of them. How is it that these bacteria are not destroyed by the immune system?

During the first three months or so of life, the infant's immune system doesn't react at all. This is known as immune tolerance. A tiny number of babies may need a liver transplant at this age but, if so, immunosuppressive drugs are not needed to prevent the new liver being rejected – the transplanted organ is accepted by the immune system as 'self', that is to say, a normal part of the infant's body. It is likely that in health the purpose of immune tolerance is to enable the baby to establish a population of bacteria in the large intestine. Those bacteria that the baby meets during that period are accepted as 'self' and survive.

When the baby is a few weeks old, however, the window of immune tolerance closes, and thereafter any bacteria that are not already recognised by the immune system as 'self' are vigorously rejected and cannot establish themselves permanently in the gut flora. This phenomenon is called 'colonisation resistance', and it means that the gut flora remains very stable during healthy adult life.

It follows that although any bacteria that the infant encounters in the early weeks of life will be regarded as normal members of bacterial flora for the rest of that individual's life, it is not possible to correct and maintain the gut flora simply by taking preparations of probiotic bacteria, whatever they may be (and despite what television advertisements may say). Unless the organism has been encountered in infancy, in health it will not colonise the gut.

Interesting indirect support for this theory was recently published. It had been shown that if mothers in late pregnancy and infants at birth were given the probiotic agent *Lactobacillus casei* GG the incidence of allergic diseases in the children during early childhood was reduced. In one study in which this probiotic was given to mothers and children for this purpose, the organism was found to disappear from the stools of the mothers as soon as they stopped taking the bacteria. In the infants, however, it was still present two years later, implying that it had become accepted as part of their normal flora, although not in those of their mothers.

COLONISATION RESISTANCE AND IBS

It seems possible that in IBS – especially caused by malfermentation – some key species of bacteria have been lost from the normal flora as a result of gastrointestinal infection or treatment with antibiotics. This leaves an empty niche that is available for further colonisation, but any bacteria that start to grow there cannot survive unless they are members of the baby's original gut flora.

This might account for the instability that we have seen in the gut flora in IBS. Different species come and go and their numbers rise and fall because, as each organism comes in, its survival is limited and it eventually disappears. These changes in the flora lead to the malfermentation of food residues which in turn produces the symptoms.

Obviously, if one knew which specific bacterium was missing, the ideal treatment would be to replace it. Probably, such replacement occurs very frequently in extended families that live together in close proximity. Children receive a very similar gut flora from the same mother and if an organism is lost because of gastrointestinal infections, it can easily be replaced by contact with siblings.

In the UK today, however, we live in small nuclear families, kept in a pristine state of cleanliness by the use of disinfectants that 'kill 99.9 per cent of all household germs'. Under these conditions of cleanliness, transmission of bacteria from one member of the family to another is clearly much less likely to happen, and damage to the gut flora more likely to persist.

PROBIOTIC BACTERIA

Nevertheless, bacteria may have beneficial effects on the bowel while they are passing along it, even if they cannot colonise the intestine and live there permanently. Probiotics are *living* bacteria that, when taken in sufficient numbers, produce health benefits beyond their simple nutritional or pharmacological value, such as relieving diarrhoea or excess flatulence. A successful probiotic organism is rather special. It must possess the following characteristics:

➤ It must not cause disease.

➤ It must not contain any toxins.

➤ It must be resistant to the effects of acid (so it can pass through the stomach without being destroyed).

➤ It must be resistant to the effects of alkalis, bile salts and digestive enzymes in the small bowel.

➤ It must be able to compete with the resident bacteria living in the lower bowel.

➤ It must be able to attach itself to the lining of the bowel so that it is not swept straight out.

➤ It should produce chemicals that repel other bacteria (known as *bacteriocins*), allowing the probiotic organism to survive in their presence.

Once in the gut, probiotic bacteria might have beneficial effects in a number of ways. As well as being of assistance in reducing fermentation in the gut, they may also suppress inflammation, help break down bile acids, reduce the secretion of mucus and fluids into the intestine, inhibit enzymes in competing bacteria or compete for bacterial nutrients, stop other bacteria attaching themselves to the lining of the gut or invading body tissues and, finally, they may repel other bacteria by the production of *bacteriocins*.

The theory that probiotic bacteria might improve health has been around for a very long time. It was the Russian Nobel Prize-winning scientist Eli Metchnikoff who first suggested that the reason that some people in central Europe were enjoying very long lives was that they were in the habit of drinking fermented milk that had been turned sour by bacteria such as *Lactobacilli* and *Bifidobacter*.

Bacteria of this sort have been widely used to make yoghurts, but the ones selected on the basis that they produced a delicious creamy yoghurt are of very little help in improving abdominal pain or diarrhoea. As the numbers of *Lactobacilli* and *Bifidobacter* have been shown to be low in IBS patients, it seemed logical that these should be the bacteria most likely to be effective probiotics. However, despite the fact that the shelves of health shops contain many strains of such bacteria called *Acidophilus*, *Super Acidophilus* and names such as these, the evidence that they were effective was sadly lacking. Furthermore, assessing their benefit in IBS is not as straightforward as it might seem. This is partly due to the nature of the condition. As there is no recognised objective abnormality to be detected in IBS, there can be no marker which can be followed to see if it is favourably influenced by the effects of probiotic bacteria. What is more a patient's symptoms may be improved by the placebo effect.

THE PLACEBO EFFECT

Patients with IBS come to the doctor complaining of symptoms for which no cause can be discovered; therefore the evaluation of treatment depends on seeing whether those symptoms improve. This unfortunately introduces a major problem, the placebo effect. Patients who have an unpleasant longstanding condition that makes their life miserable naturally want to get better as fast as they can.

If doctors suggest that they can offer a new treatment, patients' hopes are raised. They want to believe that they are getting better. We discuss in Chapter 7 how important psychological factors may be in some cases of IBS. It's not surprising that when such patients are given a new treatment, there may be a genuine short-lived improvement.

When there appears to be a physical abnormality such as malfermentation or constipation, it might seem unlikely that any genuine benefit can arise from an ineffective treatment. Nevertheless, the patients' hopes may be raised to such an extent that they believe their symptoms are less – that they are passing less wind, that their bloating is less severe or they can last longer before having to rush to the loo. This is known as the 'placebo effect'.

One example of this was shown in a study we performed to test a new agent that was hoped would relieve diarrhoea in IBS. In order to get an idea of the base line symptoms, which the patients in the trial were suffering, they were all given a three-week course of dummy tablets before being randomly assigned to an active treatment or a placebo. Unfortunately, the agent was not very effective and the trial proved to be negative. Several of our patients, however, claimed that they felt much better during the first three weeks of the trial – during the run-in period when we knew that they had all been taking a dummy! Several of them asked to be allowed to try these tablets again – even after we had explained what they were!

The influence of the placebo effect can also be seen in several of the trials of probiotics in IBS which have been published. In a number of them, symptoms in the placebo group improve in the short term, sometimes to a greater extent than those taking the active treatment. This of course may make it difficult to show that the probiotic is having any effect other than those produced by chance.

It has been estimated that the placebo response in IBS may be as high as 40 per cent, which means that symptoms are reduced to nearly half the original level by an inactive agent. This obviously makes it difficult to be sure that any beneficial effect produced by the probiotic is not simply due to this. Nevertheless, the placebo effect usually disappears after three or four weeks as the patient gradually realises that the underlying situation remains unchanged.

Therefore, trials of probiotic agents should continue for at least four weeks – ideally, for several months. Trials are also better if they are crossover, which means that the patient has a spell both on the active treatment and on the dummy so that the effects of the two can be compared in the same subject.

TRYING A PROBIOTIC

There is no perfect probiotic agent available at present. You will see many different types on the shelves of supermarkets and health stores, but there is none that can be wholeheartedly recommended for the treatment of IBS at this stage. What is more, many of them are very expensive.

Our research does suggest that there will be a role for probiotic bacteria in the management of IBS in the future. You can expect many more strains of bacteria to be tested. At present it would seem that the crucial factors for potential success include a large number of living bacteria to be administered in each dose, and that success is more likely if several different types of bacteria are used, rather than a single strain.

If you want to try probiotics, be very wary of preparations that may be recommended in shops or on television. It is absolutely essential that the bacteria they contain are alive and capable of growing in the bowel if they are to be effective and it is very difficult for the average consumer to obtain definite proof of this.

Note down your symptoms for at least two weeks before you start taking a probiotic and do this again at the end of four to five weeks to make quite sure you are benefiting before continuing with this treatment. If it does help, you will have to continue taking the bacteria indefinitely, as when you stop taking it, you will go back to square one! It would be worth a trial of one or more of the following:

➤ Lactobacillus Extra made by Lamberts in Tunbridge Wells contains both *Lactobacilli* and *Bifidobacteria* and testing has shown that the organisms are all alive and kicking and present in large numbers.

➤ *Lactobacillus casei* strain Shirota (Yakult) is easily available, but contains only a single bacterial strain. Yakult was developed in Japan early in the twentieth century and has been available in the UK for more than 10 years. In Japan it was largely regarded as something that would improve peoples' general health, and it's only recently that claims have been made about its value in IBS. Two studies, however, have now been published saying that it may have a positive effect on constipation. In both studies the frequency of defecation increased and the stools became softer. However there was little effect on other symptoms such has flatulence, pain or bloating and these patients suffered a fairly minor degree of constipation, most of them passing between three to five stools per week.

➤ Replete made by Biocare contains both *Lactobacilli* and *Bifidobacteria* and may also sometimes be helpful, but it is expensive (costing £45 for five days', treatment). In the long term this cannot be cost effective.

➤ VSL#3 can be obtained on the Internet, and is marketed in Britain by Ferring Pharmaceuticals. It is a mixture of eight different bacteria in very high numbers. There are three different *Bifidobacteria* (*B. longum, B. infantis* and *B. brevis*), four different *Lactobacilli* (*L. acidophilus, L. casei, L. bulgaricus,* and *L. plantarum*) and also *Streptococcus salivarius* sub species *thermophilus*). A single dose of VSL#3 contains no less than 450 billion organisms. There has been a great hope that it might be of value in IBS, but trials performed so far suggest that the main effect is to reduce bloating, with little effect on bowel function or pain.

This list is not meant to be comprehensive, and contains only probiotic preparations that I know some of my patients have found to be useful. There may be others that are equally good. Keep your eyes and ears open – but always remember to test a preparation's effectiveness on **your** symptoms before paying out to take it long-term. Just because someone else says that a probiotic is wonderful does not mean that it is bound to be so in your case.

PREBIOTICS

Because of the difficulties in introducing new bacteria into the intestine, attempts have been made to improve the bowel flora by feeding substances which would promote the growth of beneficial organisms such as *Bifidobacteria*. These chemicals are known as prebiotics.

Prebiotics are not digested or absorbed in the upper small intestine and therefore pass down unchanged so they can be a source of nutrition and energy for bacteria in the large intestine. Many of them are complex, or indigestible, sugars such as fructose oligosaccharide (FOS) or lactulose. The great theoretical advantage of prebiotics is that they encourage the growth of bacteria that are 'at home' in the patient's gut. Thus colonisation resistance is by-passed and any beneficial effects should be longer lasting. It has further been suggested that a mixture of probiotic bacteria and prebiotic sugars (called a synbiotic) might have even greater benefit in improving gut flora.

Interest in FOS arose when some studies showed that the number of *Bifidobacteria* in the stools of healthy volunteers increased relatively more than did the numbers of other bacteria. As these bacteria are known to be valuable lactic acid bacteria, and their numbers are reduced in IBS, it seemed that this might be a way forward to get round all the wretched problems caused by colonisation resistance, and to correct malfermentation.

However, in our experience, it is not only *Bifidobacteria* and *Lactobacilli* that flourish when supplied with prebiotics. In a controlled trial of FOS – 6 g given daily – published in 1999, we found that many IBS patients complained of an unpleasant increase in wind and discomfort – no doubt because other bacteria were increased in activity as well. Overall, there was no significant improvement in symptoms.

SUMMARY

➤ A lack of 'good' bacteria in the gut is thought to an important factor in IBS. No way has yet been found to correct this problem in adults permanently.

➤ Probiotics are 'good' bacteria added to foods such as yoghurt, or available in capsules, that may help improve gut function.

➤ Different types of probiotic bacteria are available but none has yet proved ideal for IBS sufferers and many are expensive.

➤ Some IBS sufferers do claim to benefit from taking probiotic products, however, so you may wish to try them for a trial period.

➤ Make sure the probiotic you choose contains live bacteria of the right species, such as *Bifidobacteria* or *Lactobacilli*.

➤ Note down your symptoms for two weeks before trying a probiotic and continue to monitor your symptoms for five weeks during the trial period to see if you are improving.

➤ Prebiotics are chemicals such as complex sugars that may help probiotic bacteria thrive. They can have unpleasant side effects and so far there is little evidence they work.

CHAPTER 10

The Menstrual Cycle and IBS

IBS occurs much more frequently in women than it does in men and often begins in early adult life. It's not surprising therefore that IBS may be related to changes in hormones during the menstrual cycle.

Changes in hormone levels during the menstrual cycle may produce a variety of symptoms that vary from woman to woman. Most women are cheerful and happy between the end of a period and the time of ovulation, when the hormone oestrogen has the strongest influence. After ovulation, however, oestrogen levels fall and the picture changes. Progesterone levels rise (to protect the embryo, in case conception has occurred), and the woman is more likely to suffer symptoms. Gut symptoms are very common. Many women report that they have diarrhoea or constipation just before their period starts. All these symptoms rapidly clear once the period begins.

Many women gain weight in the week before their periods due to fluid retention and this may be associated with feelings of bloatedness, with clothing being uncomfortably tight. Fluid retention may be so marked as to cause the ankles to swell. Breast symptoms can be particularly severe, with tenderness, enlargement, heaviness and pain. Other symptoms include acne and greasy hair. There may also be changes in mood and behaviour during the week before a period, including depression and decreased libido. Women are more likely to commit minor crimes at this time and suicide occurs more frequently in the week preceding menstruation. These changes may partially explain why men sometimes claim that they find women's behaviour difficult to understand at this time.

Occasionally, such symptoms in the second half of the menstrual cycle become so severe that they require medical attention. This is referred to as premenstrual syndrome (PMS). PMS is thought commonly to be triggered by stress and tension, at home or at work, and particularly affects women between the ages of 20 and 30. The behavioural changes are often extreme, with depression and tension associated with unreasonable outbursts of temper.

Gut symptoms may occur with PMS, and diarrhoea or constipation may be associated with nausea and vomiting. In most cases of PMS, symptoms arising from the gut are not a major problem. In a few cases, however, symptoms are so marked that they become the predominant feature. So there is a potential overlap between PMS and IBS.

Many women with IBS who have symptoms persistently throughout the month nevertheless report that symptoms are worse just before their periods. Symptoms may also be exacerbated shortly after ovulation, perhaps because oestrogen levels often fall markedly at that stage.

Continuing symptoms may muddy the waters and obscure a clear link between the menstrual cycle and the gut problems. Furthermore, when a woman has had a hysterectomy, it is usual to leave the ovaries in place. The hormonal changes of the menstrual cycle then continue, even though the removal of the uterus means that periods cease. The link between the menstrual cycle and symptoms thus may be even more obscure and it may be necessary to complete a symptom diary over two months or so, to confirm that the gut symptoms are associated with changes that may be hormone induced, such as weight gain, bloating and breast tenderness.

EXAGGERATED GUT EFFECTS

Therefore hormone changes during the cycle may be a cause of IBS. Many people would consider that this was due simply to psychological factors. Women tend to be anxious and upset before their periods and this can lead to symptoms in the gut. Disordered breathing patterns (see page 98) become worse at this time. However, it is not at all clear that such a psychological explanation is indeed true. The mechanism of PMS remains uncertain. The condition has been difficult to study because these symptoms vary so much from woman to woman, which makes it difficult to be exactly sure who has PMS and who merely has an exaggeration of the normal effects of the menstrual cycle.

Various theories have been put forward concerning the balance between oestrogen and progesterone, excessive production of prolactin, or of hormones that may affect the function of the kidneys. None of these has been substantiated. One of the few facts that is indisputable is that PMS disappears if the ovaries are removed.

The overlap between PMS and IBS and the important role that we have demonstrated for the gut bacteria in IBS has led to the suggestion that the gut bacteria might also have a role to play in PMS. I suggested this in a lecture to the National Association for Premenstrual Syndrome in Birmingham 1995. Put simply, the theory suggests that progesterone may increase the activity of the gut bacteria during the second half of the menstrual cycle. This might produce symptoms in just the same way as increased bacterial activity leads to malfermentation in some cases of IBS (see Chapter 5). Little research has been done to test this theory. For example, no one has ever shown that the bacteria living in the bowel in women with PMS are any different from those in other women.

TREATMENT OF MENSTRUALLY-RELATED IBS

It's clear that it's sometimes difficult to make a distinction between IBS and PMS. Indeed, menstrually-related IBS may simply be PMS with gut symptoms that are more prominent than is usual. Like IBS, the treatment of PMS has been unsatisfactory. Pyridoxine (vitamin B6) is the simplest treatment in PMS and helps many women. It is customary to recommend taking 100 mg daily, but doubts have been raised about the safety of this and nowadays 50 mg daily is more usual. Fluid retention and weight gain may be reduced by taking tablets called diuretics that increase the flow of urine.

As both PMS and menstrually-related IBS are clearly affected by hormone changes, it seems logical to try manipulating hormone levels in the hope of improving symptoms. Hormones related to progesterone have long been advocated for the treatment of PMS, but no convincing physiological basis for this has ever been shown. As the whole point of the present book is to demonstrate that IBS can be satisfactorily managed if the physiological principles underlying its causes are understood, it is only sensible that the treatment recommended for menstrually-related IBS should also be based on such principles, and so therapy based on progesterone will not be considered further.

In younger women, the most practical approach in the management of menstrually-related IBS is to use oral contraceptives. These reduce the level of ovarian hormones so that the effects of the menstrual cycle are much less acute. Blood loss and period pain is reduced and IBS symptoms related to the gut are often considerably improved. In older women, hormone replacement therapy (HRT) may be more suitable and this again is something you should discuss with your doctor. In women beyond the menopause, IBS related to hormone changes usually settles completely.

If menstrually-related IBS is indeed related to changes in the activity of the colonic bacteria, it should also be possible to control it by diet. Again, controlled trials are lacking, but a number of books have been written that recommend diets to control symptoms arising pre-menstrually, and these diets are usually very similar to the exclusion diet that we have described earlier (see page 66).

If you prefer not to try hormonal methods of controlling your symptoms, or if they don't work, it would be well worthwhile trying the exclusion diet. If you find you have food intolerances, it may only be necessary to avoid the foods in question during the week preceding your period.

Many gynaecologists have special experience in manipulating hormonal changes during the menstrual cycle, and it may be well worth seeking such advice if menstrually related IBS proves difficult to control.

SUMMARY

➤ Many women find that IBS symptoms occur or get worse just before their period.

➤ Increased progesterone may boost bacterial activity in the bowel leading to malfermentation (see page 53), but this theory remains unproven.

➤ If IBS symptoms are linked to the menstrual cycle, younger women may benefit from taking oral contraceptives, and post-menopausal women from HRT.

➤ Alternatively, an exclusion diet may help to identify problem foods that should then be excluded from the diet during the week before your period.

CHAPTER 11

Musculo-Skeletal Causes of Abdominal Pain

Many patients are told they have IBS when there is nothing wrong with their gut at all. This is because many busy doctors carry around in their minds the simple equation:

Abdominal pain + nothing wrong in the gut = IBS.

In fact, abdominal pain can easily arise from causes **outside** the gut. We saw in the previous chapter what a large overlap there may be with gynaecological problems in women. Abdominal pain may also arise from damage to the muscles of the abdominal wall and the nerves and bones that supply and support it. Of course, this sort of problem would never fit the precise definition of IBS provided by the Rome Criteria (page 9). Nevertheless, many patients are sent to specialist gastroenterologists for investigation of bowel pain that is subsequently shown to be the result of such musculo-skeletal causes.

In one study at Addenbrooke's hospital, out of 200 patients referred for investigation of abdominal pain who were reviewed by a specialist physiotherapist, no fewer than 19 were found to have pain arising from a musculo-skeletal cause. So, if you scored highly in the musculo-skeletal section of the questionnaire in Chapter 3, read on...It's very likely that you will find a solution to your problem.

CAUSES OF MUSCULO-SKELETAL ABDOMINAL PAIN

These pains are caused by:

➤ Trapped spinal nerves.

➤ Trapped abdominal nerves.

➤ Torn fibres in the abdominal muscles.

TRAPPED SPINAL NERVES

Back problems are so common that they are one of the most important reasons for loss of time from work in the UK today. The spine is made up of a column of bones called the spinal vertebrae, piled up like bricks set one on top of another. Anyone who has watched a young child playing with bricks will appreciate how unstable such a tower may become. Much of the weight of the body is suspended from the spine and balanced, sometimes precariously, on just two legs for support. So it's little wonder that problems sometimes arise. Back problems are usually due to repeated misuse of the back and failure to keep the supporting muscles strong and supple.

Nerves leave the spine from between each building block (or vertebra), and run to all parts of the body. It's well known that pressure on these nerves by displaced spinal bones or joints may lead to pain in the area that the nerves supply, but this principle is rarely applied to the abdomen. Just as in sciatica, where a nerve in the lower spine is compressed producing pain down the back of the leg, which may run even into the toes, so trapped nerves may lead to pain in the abdominal wall.

TRAPPED ABDOMINAL NERVES

Nerves may also become trapped follow abdominal surgery. When surgeons make an incision they inevitably cut through the nerves that supply the abdominal wall. Usually after surgery these heal perfectly satisfactorily, but sometimes they do not. They may become trapped in scar tissue and this can lead to a painful nodule called a neuroma.

TORN MUSCLE FIBRES

Muscle tears are usually the result of injury. Abdominal muscles are of crucial importance in stabilising the upper body. Though we are often unaware of their importance, they work very hard when we are exercising and particularly when we are lifting. Sudden and unexpected exertion may exceed the strength of the muscles, which may then tear. Such a tear may give rise to chronic pain.

The matter may be further complicated because if muscle fibres are torn from their connections to the ribs or the connective tissues that anchor them, chronic inflammation may arise, producing a tiny inflammatory nodule, sometimes referred to as a myofascial nodule. One of the best known examples of this is tennis elbow. In this, fibres of one of the strongest muscles in the forearm (*brachio-radialis*) may be torn from its bony anchor in the upper arm. This classically occurs, of course, while playing tennis, but other similar exertion may have just the same effect on any muscle – including in the abdomen – if it is not strong enough to meet the demands placed upon it. The nodule of torn muscle fibres may become inflamed and lead to chronic pain and discomfort that goes on for many months or even years.

There are two common sites for this sort of nodule to form in the abdomen:

➤ At the point where the muscles attach to the lower ribs (sometimes called the 'slipping-rib' syndrome).

➤ Where the muscles join the rectus sheath – a band of tissue that separates the powerful 'six-pack' muscle at the very front of the abdomen (*rectus abdominis*) with the muscles on the side of the abdomen. A tear at this point often produces an inflammatory nodule.

Sometimes, however, abdominal pain arises simply because there seems to be an imbalance in the strength and efficiency of one group of abdominal muscles as opposed to another leading to compensation elsewhere, displacement and, eventually, chronic discomfort.

CASE STUDY

A typical example of how muscle injury can cause abdominal pain was the case of a woman of 45 who was sent first to gynaecologists and then to a gastro-enterologist for investigation for pain in her lower abdomen. She had gone through all sorts of normal investigations before the story emerged of how, while going up into her loft to hunt for a discarded suitcase, she had stepped in the wrong place and one leg had gone right through the ceiling into the bedroom below. She sat down with a nasty bump. With hindsight, it was apparent that it was after this accident that her pain started. The pain was caused by muscle tears and when she was referred for appropriate physiotherapy, her symptoms rapidly cleared.

HOW TO SPOT A MUSCULO-SKELETAL PAIN

If you scored highly on the musculo-skeletal section of our questionnaire it's quite likely that your pain is at least in part caused by musculo-skeletal factors. Before thinking about any treatment, however, you may like to consider the following factors and see how well they apply to your case.

➤ Musculo-skeletal pains do not arise in the gut and there is therefore no upset of gut function (unless, of course, other factors are also in play). Bowel function is normal and the pain is not affected by meals. Some people have claimed that their pains were worse after their evening meals, but this may merely reflect the fact that the pain gets more severe as the day wears on. If the pain is due to musculo-skeletal causes only, eating in the morning will not cause any difficulty and there will be no excess wind or bloating.

➤ Musculo-skeletal pains get worse as the day gets on and the patient becomes more tired.

➤ Often musculo-skeletal pains can be provoked by exertion such as lifting, bending, twisting or even just rolling over in bed. In general, though, because the patient is resting, the pain does not get worse in bed at night and has usually cleared on waking in the morning.

➤ Musculo-skeletal pain often spreads elsewhere, particularly if caused by a trapped nerve. Typically, this may be to the back, but sometimes it spreads to the leg as well. Pain that spreads to the leg is never caused by genuine IBS.

CONFIRMATORY TESTS

If it seems likely that your pain is musculo-skeletal, try the following tests:

1. Lie on your bed on your back, fold your arms across your chest and sit up just using the muscles of the abdominal wall to pull you upright. If this makes the pain worse, it is very likely to be arising from the muscles of the abdominal wall.

2. Still lying on your back on the bed, roll over from one side to another, twisting your spine. If this makes the pain worse, it again suggests that the cause is musculo-skeletal.

3. Try coughing as hard as you can. If the pain is musculo-skeletal you will usually find that this makes it worse, as does sneezing.

HOW IS MUSCULO-SKELETAL PAIN TREATED?

In the first instance, and certainly in mild cases, a little self-help may provide a great deal of relief.

SIMPLE PAINKILLERS

Doctors divide pain into two types: visceral pain and somatic pain. Visceral pains arise in the gut and other internal organs and usually require strong painkillers derived from morphine. Somatic pains arise from the limbs, joints and muscles and respond to simpler measures such as paracetamol and ibuprofen. If your pain is eased by paracetamol or ibuprofen it is probably musculo-skeletal. The pain of true IBS, which arises from the gut, is unaffected by them.

REST

It is obviously sensible to rest the muscle that is painful to see if this hastens its recovery.

SUPPORT

Check your bed to see if it's providing adequate support for your spine. If it's an old bed, it may have become too soft and may sag in the middle. While you are thinking about replacing it with a more suitable option, it is worthwhile placing a board between the mattress and the base. For a double bed, this should be wide enough to stretch across both sides and extend from your shoulders down below the level of your bottom.

PHYSIOTHERAPY

If the pain persists, despite these simple measures, you should consult your GP. Explain that you think the pains in your stomach could be musculo-skeletal rather than being caused by IBS and say why you think this is the case. For example, say the pain gets worse after certain muscular actions and that your gut appears to be functioning perfectly. You may then be referred to a physiotherapist. Failing this you can always make an appointment privately to see a physiotherapist or an osteopath.

A physiotherapist will work, firstly, to relieve the pain and, secondly, to stretch and strengthen the muscles that are affected, to prevent the problem returning in the long term.

The Role of the Physiotherapist

The physiotherapist will assess you from a musculo-skeletal point of view. He or she will examine the spine looking at posture, spinal mobility and areas of stiffness. The abdomen will be assessed for strength of muscles and any areas of tenderness and/or myofascial nodules. Treatment is based on their findings and usually includes two elements:

➤ ***Local treatment:*** *This can include application of heat, massage, mobilisations and ultrasound to areas of pain and tenderness. Ultrasound has been found to be very effective in the treatment of inflammatory/myofascial nodules. It helps to reduce inflammation and break up fibrous connections and therefore reduce pain.*

➤ ***Exercises/posture and stretches:*** *An individualised programme of exercises will be given to improve strength and mobility, making sure there is a good balance between the back and abdominal muscles. Posture is addressed as often this is poor in the person who has had long-term abdominal pain. In response to abdominal pain we tend to flex forwards, allowing the lower back to over-stretch and the abdominal muscles to 'bunch' up. This can affect the movement of the layers of abdominal muscles on one another. In such cases, the physiotherapist will give specific stretching exercises.*

A combination of local treatment and a specific exercise programme can relieve the pain. The exercises that you are given are very important and it is essential that you follow them conscientiously. Even if your symptoms go away completely, it is best to continue your exercises long term to prevent a re-occurrence.

You will also be advised on the correct way to lift. It is necessary at all times to keep your back straight so that the weight is not carried by the joints between the vertebrae of the spine but by the powerful muscles of the thighs. To lift something heavy, bend your knees and squat down and then lift the object keeping your back straight. This should become your unfailing practice.

If, despite all these measures, musculo-skeletal pain persists, further specialist measures may be necessary. Your doctor may decide to refer you to a rheumatologist, particularly if he/she believes there is a problem with the spine. Alternatively your doctor may wish to refer you to a pain clinic (see below). The possible value of an exclusion diet is also discussed below.

Pain Clinics

Clinics that specialise in pain control are now very popular and exist in most large hospitals in the UK. When a specific nerve pathway can be shown to be transmitting a pain, anaesthetising it or destroying it (a nerve-block) may prove of enormous value. So far, however, pain clinics have not featured strongly in this book. It's my belief that there is virtually no role at all for them in the management of gastrointestinal disease, except sometimes to destroy ganglia, through which nerves carrying painful impulses pass, in cases of terminal gastrointestinal cancer.

The pathways of pain from the gut to the brain are very complex and therefore such nerve blocks are not applicable to patients with IBS. When those suffering from unexplained gut pain are referred to a pain clinic, they are frequently offered little more than psycho-

logical counselling and an anti-depressant. If these measures worked this book would not be necessary.

However, as musculo-skeletal pains do not arise from the gut, the pain clinic may be very helpful. In particular, inflammatory nodules may be injected with a mixture of hydrocortisone and local anaesthetic to produce considerable relief if not a complete cure. Indeed, such injections may be given by your gastro-enterologist or by your GP. Injections into the complex joints of the spine can also be helpful and as these need x-ray facilities to ensure they hit the right spot, then of course they are a job for a specialist from the pain clinic.

EXCLUSION DIETS

Over the years, I have encountered a few patients with apparent musculo-skeletal abdominal pains who found their symptoms were resolved completely by an exclusion diet when all other measures had failed. Unfortunately I am not clear on the mechanisms by which an exclusion diet proves effective. It may be akin to its action in rheumatoid arthritis in that it reduces swelling of joint tissues, thus relieving pain. Some of my patients have found consistent relief for many years and the pain returns if they slip up on the diet and eat the wrong things.

Wheat is the commonest food involved and as it is very inconvenient to exclude wheat from the diet, it is generally best to keep an exclusion diet for those cases that have not responded to simpler measures. The diet should be tried for three weeks and if there is no benefit at the end of that time, the patient must return to normal eating. If the symptoms clear, then food should be reintroduced as described in Chapter 5.

SUMMARY

➤ Injury to the spine, spinal nerves, abdominal nerves or abdominal muscles can lead to musculo-skeletal pain that may mimic IBS symptoms.

➤ If this is the cause, the pain will probably increase during the day and get much worse when you sit up or turn over in bed.

➤ If abdominal pain is eased by paracetamol or ibuprofen it is musculo-skeletal – not IBS.

➤ Rest and painkillers are the simplest self-help measures to take.

➤ If these don't work, a doctor may refer you to a physiotherapist for heat treatment and an exercise programme.

➤ In difficult cases, a pain clinic may help.

➤ An exclusion diet can be effective in rare cases, but why is unclear.

CHAPTER 12

What If You're Still No Better?

If you have reached this stage in the book, and have worked through the various causes that are known to produce IBS, and yet you are still not any better, you'll be feeling very disappointed. Do not despair! There are a number of other conditions that produce symptoms similar to IBS and yet which cannot be called IBS because of the distinct but subtle physical problems that underlie them.

You may think that these conditions should have been excluded during the first medical tests when the doctors were checking you out. Conditions that mimic IBS, however, are not usually detected from a routine medical history and examination, nor by the battery of tests that are recommended to exclude organic causes. They need special tests to pick them up and there is no way we can teach you how to deal with them in a self-help book.

However, we are going to go through some of the most important conditions here, so that if you find that your symptoms don't fit into any of the established causes of IBS, you can discuss with your doctor whether it may be worthwhile checking for them, in the hope that you find a satisfactory way to deal with your problem.

BILE SALT MALABSORPTION

If you are suffering from chronic diarrhoea without pain, it may be worthwhile discussing with your doctor whether or not you should be investigated for bile salt malabsorption. Bile salts are produced in the liver and secreted in the bile. They are very important in the digestion of fatty foods. As everyone knows who has tossed a salad, oil and water do not mix. In a salad dressing the olive oil keeps separating from the vinegar. The contents of the gut are watery and the fat in the food cannot easily be dissolved in order that it may be accessible for digestion to fat-splitting enzymes – it needs to be emulsified. Bile salts provide the mechanism for this.

They are complex molecules, one end of which will dissolve in water and the other end in fat. When they come into contact with water, they form microscopic little clusters called micelles with the water-soluble end of the molecules on the outside so that the micelle can dissolve easily. As the water-soluble ends are all on the outside, it follows that the fat-soluble ends are all on the inside, providing a space in which fats can easily be carried and where they can be digested by fat-splitting enzymes and the products of digestion absorbed.

Bile salts are therefore very important and very precious. The bile containing them is stored in the gallbladder, which contracts when a meal containing fat is eaten. Bile passes out into the duodenum (the first part of the small intestine) where it emulsifies the fats ready for digestion. When the fats have been digested and absorbed, the bile salts remain in the intestine and would be expected to pass out with other food residues. However, at the very end of the small intestine, in a region called the terminal ileum, there is a short region only a few centimetres long where special cells reabsorb the bile salts.

Once back in the blood they are recycled, going back to the liver and being secreted once more in the bile. This recycling process is highly efficient. The body usually contains 2–4 g of bile acids that undergo this circulation five to 10 times each day. Less than half a gram per day escapes reabsorption and passes into the large intestine.

Bile salts that reach the large intestine may cause an increased secretion of fluid and if this is excessive it may lead to diarrhoea. Damage to the specialised reabsorbing cells at the end of the small intestine may be caused by a number of diseases such as Crohn's disease, bacterial overgrowth in the intestine and, of course, if that part of the intestine has been removed by surgery, it is no longer available to reabsorb them. The re-uptake of bile salts can be reduced for no obvious reason – a condition called idiopathic bile salt malabsorption. This can be detected quite easily by a test called the selenium-75-homocholic acid taurine test, usually abbreviated to SeHCAT.

SeHCAT is an artificial bile salt labelled with a tiny amount of selenium-75. Patients are given a small oral dose and when it has been absorbed, the total radiation given off by the body is determined. A week later the patient returns to the clinic and the whole body radiation is determined again. By calculating how much radiation has been lost from the body during the week, it is possible to calculate what percentage of the bile salt remains.

If the test shows excessive losses of bile salts, it means that they are not adequately being reabsorbed. It is then fairly simple to control the diarrhoea by giving resins that bind bile salts. These resins, such as cholestyramine and colestipol, prevent the bile salts coming into contact with the lining of the large intestine, and so reduce the amount of diarrhoea. Alternatively, it may suffice to give a simple anti-diarrhoea drug such as Loperamide.

ENTERIC NEUROPATHY

In this condition there is damage to the nerves that supply the gut (the enteric nervous system). This means that the process of peristalsis (the smooth flow of food and waste along the gut) is disrupted. The small bowel contains very large amounts of nutrients in the foods that are being digested. These provide an excellent medium for the growth of bacteria. In health, however, the small bowel does not contain bacteria because its contents are slightly alkaline and contain powerful digestive enzymes that make it a hostile place for bacteria to survive.

Even more importantly, peristalsis normally sweeps the contents of the gut along so efficiently that bacteria never have the opportunity to establish themselves. If the small bowel is diseased and becomes dilated or narrowed, however, the flow of food along the gut becomes sluggish. Under these circumstances, bacteria can colonise the small intestine and live on the nutrients passing along it. This sort of problem can usually be picked up very readily by x-rays of the small intestine.

In patients with enteric neuropathies, however, there is no damage to the gut itself and an x-ray will appear quite normal. Disruption of the normal process of peristalsis nevertheless leads to a sluggish flow so that bacteria can establish themselves even though the calibre of the bowel is unchanged. When bacteria come into contact with food, they ferment it.

The single commonest cause of true IBS is the fermentation of food residues leaving the small gut by abnormal bacteria in the large bowel (Chapter 5). Problems arise in a similar way when bacteria get into the wrong place – as in the small intestine. Once again the result is malfermentation and the symptoms suffered by patients with an enteric neuropathy are very similar to those of IBS including pain, wind, bloating and diarrhoea.

Unlike IBS, however, the malfermentation of an enteric neuropathy does not respond to diet. This is because the diets used in IBS are based on those foods that by and large are completely digested in the small intestine and thus provide little residue for the bacteria of the large intestine to work on. Bacteria that live in the small intestine are able to ferment food before it has been digested fully, whatever type of diet the patient is eating. Thus dietary measures are of little help. As at present there is no known way of restoring the function of the damaged nerve fibres, the best line of treatment is to kill off the bacteria in the small bowel by suitable antibiotics.

The diagnosis of an enteric neuropathy is not easy. Complete proof depends on the detection of abnormal patterns of small intestine contraction and this is a complex procedure in which pressure monitors must be swallowed and guided down into the small intestine. Such a test is only available in specialised hospitals.

It is, however, quite simple to establish that there are bacteria growing in the small intestine. As we saw in Chapter 5, when bacteria ferment food residues, they release hydrogen that can be measured on the breath. It is possible to adapt this for diagnostic purposes by giving patients different sugars that are broken down in different parts of the intestine.

➤ **Lactulose.** This sugar cannot be digested in the human small intestine and therefore passes through to the bacteria in the large intestine, which get to work on it, producing hydrogen. People with IBS therefore release more hydrogen after lactulose, than do others.

➤ **Lactose,** the sugar found in milk, is normally digested and completely absorbed in the small intestine, but in the condition called alactasia the enzyme to digest it disappears from the small intestine after childhood, so that drinking milk leads to pain, wind and diarrhoea in affected adults. Those affected will release more hydrogen after a drink of this sugar, whereas in normal individuals it is completely digested and no hydrogen comes off.

➤ **Glucose** is a very simple sugar that should be quickly absorbed high in the small intestine – with no hydrogen released. To check for bacteria in the small bowel we give a drink of glucose. If bacteria have colonised the small intestine, glucose will reach them before it can be absorbed and the resulting hydrogen will be detected on the breath.

If a glucose hydrogen breath test is positive, most gastroenterologists would want to do an x-ray of the small intestine, to make sure that there is no organic disease such as jejunal diverticulosis or Crohn's disease. However, such x-rays, as we have said, look normal in enteric neuropathies.

They may also wish to see exactly which bacteria are living in the small intestine. This can be done by endoscopy – a gastroscope (viewing tube) is passed down the throat into the stomach and as far along the duodenum as it will reach. A sterile tube is then passed through the gastroscope and yet further along the bowel. Small intestinal juices are sucked up and sent for culture in the laboratory.

Isolation of the bacteria concerned is important because if antibiotic treatment is to be successful, the doctor needs to choose the correct antibiotics to deal with the bacteria concerned. Bacteria may easily become resistant to some antibiotics. If the antibiotic resistance to the bacteria is known, one can be selected that is more likely to prove effective. As long-term antibiotic treatment is necessary to keep these bacteria under control, your doctor will often advise you to rotate three or four different antibiotics in turn to reduce the chances of the bacteria becoming resistant to them.

GALLBLADDER DISORDERS

IBS symptoms may be mimicked by disorders of the small intestine that generally produce diarrhoea, wind and pain. Unusual disorders of the gallbladder may also mimic IBS, but in these cases pain is the predominant problem. Patients with gallbladder disorders frequently suffer from nausea and belching and their symptoms are worse after a fatty meal.

The most important clue to gallbladder problems is the nature of the pain. Gallbladder pain is frequently quite typical. Many people know that the gallbladder is just below the ribs on the right hand side of the abdomen and expect that is where they would feel any gallbladder pain. In truth, pain in the gallbladder arises in the centre of the upper abdomen, between the breastbone and the navel. Lots of other pain such as that from an ulcer, acid reflux or pancreatic problems may be felt here too. What makes gallbladder pain different is that it spreads from the centre along the margins of the lower ribs – both sides – and also spreads to the back, typically to the shoulder blades and sometimes to the right shoulder.

This pain usually comes on after eating, particularly a fatty meal, because that's what makes the gallbladder contract and causes the pain to come on. At the same time the patient may feel sick and frequently belches. Why belching is so typical of gallbladder disease is not clear. As we have seen in Chapter 7, belching is usually the result of swallowing air and there is nothing to suggest that this occurs more frequently in people with gallbladder problems. It has been suggested that reflux of bile and pancreatic secretions into the stomach may result in stomach acid causing the release of carbon dioxide from bicarbonate, which is present in the pancreatic juice.

By far the most common source of gallbladder pain is gallstones, the pain being caused by stones temporarily blocking the duct that leads from the gallbladder to the duodenum. If an ultrasound is performed and gallstones are discovered, then the problem is usually easily resolved.

Not infrequently, however, patients with gallbladder pain have a normal ultrasound with no stones visible at all. It is not uncommon for gallstones to be overlooked on scans and sometimes, when suspicions are very strong, it may be justified to do a repeat examination. Even if gallstones are finally excluded however, there are three further possibilities which should be considered:

➤ Adenomyomatosis.

➤ Billiary dyskinesia.

➤ Sphincter of Oddi Dysfunction (SOD.)

All three of these conditions may cause biliary pain. Adenomyomatosis is a long and complicated term meaning chronic inflammation of the wall of the gallbladder with the formation of little pockets within it. In these pockets are tiny gallstones that may escape into the cavity of the gallbladder and then pass along the bile duct causing considerable discomfort. These stones can easily be demonstrated when the gallbladder has been removed, but are too small to be detected by ultrasound scanning.

Biliary dyskinesia means that the gallbladder does not contract properly. After a meal it starts to contract, but instead of expelling the bile as it should, the neck goes into spasm and on x-rays it appears as a round ball full of bile that remains where it was in the gallbladder instead of passing out into the intestine.

It is possible to give special radioisotope labelled dyes that collect in the gallbladder. If the gallbladder is then made to contract by giving a fatty food (such as a Mars Bar!) the relative amount of bile expelled into the gut can be measured and this is called the ejection fraction. If the ejection fraction is below 40 per cent, there is usually some biliary dyskinesia. Although various drugs have been tried to get the gallbladder to contract more smoothly, in most cases the best treatment is to remove it.

Finally, the sphincter of Oddi is the valve that regulates the flow of bile and pancreatic juices from the bile duct into the duodenum. If it goes into spasm preventing the passage of these fluids, then biliary pain results. This may be associated with an increase in the level in the blood of enzymes secreted by the liver or pancreas. It is possible to measure the pressure in the sphincter of Oddi by passing a little catheter up through the opening of the bile duct during endoscopy and measuring it directly. However, this is a specialised procedure that is available in only a few hospitals. Morphine will make the sphincter of Oddi contract and this is the basis of a test combined with scanning to determine the size of the obstructed duct or the rate of bile flow. It may be possible to relieve these spasms by cutting through the sphincter using an endoscope.

DISORDERS OF THE PANCREAS

Pancreatic disease may be difficult to detect in its early stages. It typically causes pain in the centre of the upper abdomen radiating to the back and made worse by eating. This may be associated with weight loss and diarrhoea and in later stages the stools contain an excess of fat. As the pancreas also produces insulin, diabetes mellitus may also occur.

Full investigation is complex and must be left to a specialist gastroenterologist. A simple test, however, to screen for pancreatic function is to check for faecal elastase. This is a pancreatic enzyme that passes out in the stools, and whose activity can therefore be determined in the laboratory. Your GP may well be able to send a sample of faeces to your local hospital for this test, if he or she believes that it is possible that your diarrhoea is caused by problems in the pancreas.

DIVERTICULAR DISEASE

Diverticula are small protrusions through the wall of the large intestine. They are thought to be yet another manifestation of a degree of constipation – a diet low in fibre produces small hard stools, which require more pressure from the muscles in the gut wall to help them along. The pressure inside the bowel rises, leading to diverticula protruding through at weak spots – such as where a blood vessel passes through. In themselves they are harmless, and they are very common in people who are middle-aged and older. They may cause trouble if they become infected (diverticulitis) or if they bleed.

They are often found in the routine investigation of people who have IBS, and their main importance is that they confirm without any doubt that the diet has been inadequate in roughage. People with diverticula feel better if they follow a high-fibre diet – unless of course they also suffer excessive flatulence, pain and bloating. If so they should chose a low fermentable fibre diet, and increase roughage with a non-fermentable bulking agent.

SUMMARY

➤ If none of the measures suggested so far have helped, your problem may be due to a less common disorder that mimics the symptoms of IBS.

➤ These include bile salt malabsorption, enteric neuropathy, disorders of the gallbladder, disorders of the pancreas and diverticular disease.

➤ These disorders all need specialist investigation and treatment.

CHAPTER 13

Continuing Control of IBS

For many years IBS has presented an apparently impenetrable jungle thick with claims and counter claims, theories and conflicts, which has frustrated the medical profession and left millions of patients in continuing misery. This problem only started to be solved once we could discern, through the jungle, the outlines of the different conditions that together make up IBS and to start a logical approach to their management. These conditions can be further examined and refined and it may well be that as each is clarified, it will allow the discovery of further causes of IBS that are still currently unsuspected. After all, we still only claim to be able to relieve satisfactorily the symptoms of 70–80 per cent of our patients. There must be more to follow.

The end of the struggle against IBS will appear when our understanding of the abnormal processes underlying the different causes of IBS gives rise to specific objective tests that can confirm the diagnosis in a way that is far more reliable than merely analysing the symptoms. The discovery that some patients with IBS produce large quantities of hydrogen suggests a possible diagnostic test. Indeed, the measurement of hydrogen excreted on the breath after administering a non-absorbable sugar like lactulose has been proposed by researchers in Los Angeles as a useful test. We disagree, as when hydrogen production is much increased, the amount excreted on the breath no longer accurately reflects total production.

Nevertheless, we believe that refinements of this technology will soon provide an objective way to confirm malfermentation. Likewise, an instrument that has been developed to measure breathing rates and the amount of carbon dioxide in the expired air seems likely to provide a way of diagnosing anxiety and air swallowing more reliably than the Nijmegen questionnaire (see page 10).

It will be a little while before the scientific studies to confirm the reliability of this as a diagnostic tool is proven, but light is visible at the end of the tunnel. When a reliable test exists for a type of IBS, it will become a separate condition and will be diagnosed and treated quite straightforwardly – as, for example, has hypolactasia. We can eventually hope that the term 'IBS' will disappear completely! The 'beginning of the end' of IBS may not yet quite be in sight, but we have surely reached the 'end of the beginning'!

You, the individual suffering from IBS, have also reached the end of the beginning. I shall be very disappointed if, having followed the plans explained in this book, you do not now understand the processes that lead to your IBS symptoms and have begun to control them in a sensible manner in order to relieve your problems. IBS is no longer a bizarre and incomprehensible condition. The principle underlying its successful management is the same as that of any other disease – find the cause and treat it logically.

Nevertheless, even though your symptoms may now be well controlled, they will return if you give up and go back to your original way of life. Many patients find that food intolerances slowly disappear as months pass by, but some have to continue dietary exclusions for many years. Similarly, patients who have retrained their breathing must continue the exercises on a regular daily basis if they are not to fall back into their bad old ways when they are under stress.

Patients who have suffered from IBS have demonstrated quite clearly that they have very sensitive guts, and it will be necessary to keep an intelligent eye open for problems in the future. If symptoms return, you should now know enough about the potential causes to be able to work out for yourself what may have gone wrong and to deal with it appropriately. If necessary, because symptoms persist, you can go back to the questionnaires in Chapter 3 and see if any new factors are responsible for a relapse in your symptoms.

A common cause of IBS is gastroenteritis and it is sensible for you to try and avoid this as much as possible. Of course, episodes of food poisoning do happen and you are as likely to get one from a meal prepared in a top restaurant, as you are from one in a greasy spoon café. If you are so unfortunate as to get gastroenteritis, stop eating solid foods until the symptoms clear and concentrate on drinking as much clear liquid as possible. This will reduce the likelihood of developing further food intolerances.

Prevention, of course, is better than cure and if you are travelling on business or holiday to a country where food poisoning is common, it's sensible to eat only freshly cooked food that is hot enough to kill off any bacteria present. You should never drink the local tap water (that includes the ice in drinks, as freezing does not kill the micro-organisms that cause disease.)

Cold dishes such as salads, ice-creams and puddings can easily be contaminated by flies and must be avoided. Avoid the lovely displays of exotic fruit set out in the smart tropical hotels and restaurants as flies will have probably crawled all over them! The inside of fruit is usually sterile, but in the Indian sub-continent, where fruit is sold by weight, dirty water may be injected to increase weights – and profits. Normally, though, if you peel fruit yourself, it should be safe.

Antibiotic treatment may cause IBS, as we have seen. It's important that you only take antibiotics when there is a very good reason for doing so – don't be persuaded to take them just to see if they may possibly do some good! We have recently published a paper showing that antibiotics used to treat infections by *Helicobacter pylori* (which causes stomach ulcers) temporarily change the gut bacteria in the same way that is seen in cases of IBS caused by malfermentation. In most cases, these changes spontaneously go back to normal.

However, the exciting development is that administration of a probiotic containing *Lactobacilli* and *Bifidobacteria* prevented this change occurring. If this work is confirmed, it suggests that it will always be sensible to protect the gut flora by taking a probiotic preparation at the same time as any antibiotic treatment.

The outlook for IBS patients is good. Many patients find that avoiding those foods that upset them becomes second nature. When asked, they forget they are following a diet. Likewise, a bulking agent or relaxation and diaphragmatic breathing become such a routine that they are no longer a handicap. You will become used to enjoying good health, and the whole vicious spiral of anxiety and distress will slowly unwind. Don't forget, however, to keep open a weather eye for problems in your gut. New symptoms must not be ignored. If they include 'red flag' danger symptoms (see page 10), consult your doctor. If they do not, consider whether they could be a new manifestation of your IBS and, if so, what would be the best way to handle them.

We know from repeated surveys, and from re-encountering patients treated many years before, that the majority of patients who approach IBS in the way explained in this book keep control of it in the long term. As the years go by, setbacks produce symptoms that are less and less severe until eventually they disappear completely. The future is bright. Whatever you do, never forget that there is a logical explanation for the symptoms of IBS, and that you have the knowledge to sort them out. Good luck!

Further Information

FURTHER READING

Camilleri M, and Spiller R C, eds, *Irritable Bowel Syndrome diagnosis and treatment*, W B Saunders, Edinburgh, 2002.

Chudleigh V, and Hunter J O, 'Chapter 41: Food allergy and intolerance' in Bosch, Hawkey, and Weinstein, eds, **Clinical Gastroenterology and Hepatology; the modern clinician's guide**, Elsevier, Edinburgh, 2005.

Chudleigh V, and Hunter J O, Chapter 23, pages 429–441, 'Diseases of the Gastrointestinal tract' in Giesler C and Powers H, eds, **Human Nutrition and Dietetics** (11th edn), Elsevier, Edinburgh, 2005.

Hunter J O, Workman E M, and Woolner J, *Solve your Food Intolerance*, Vermilion, London, 2005

USEFUL WEBSITES

General Information
www.ibsessentials.co.uk

Physiotherapy:
www.physiohypervent.org

Emotional freedom technique (EFT):
www.emofree.com

Linden Method:
www.thelindenmethod.co.uk

Bibliography

CHAPTER 3

Alun Jones V, Shorthouse M, McLaughlan P, Workman E, and Hunter J O, 'Food Intolerance: A major factor in the pathogenesis of Irritable Bowel Syndrome', **Lancet** (1982) ii: 1115-1117.

Ragnarsson G, and Bodemar G, 'Division of the irritable bowel syndrome into subgroups on the basis of daily recorded symptoms in two outpatients samples', **Scand. J Gastro** (1999) 34; 993-1000

Hunter J O, 'Hypothesis. Food Allergy or enterometabolic disorder?', **Lancet** (1991) 338; 495-496

Van Dixhoorn J, and Duivenvoorden H J, 'Efficacy of Nijmegen Questionnaire in recognition of the Hyper-ventilation Syndrome', **J Psychosom. Res.** (1985) 29; 199-206

CHAPTER 5

King T S, Elia M, and Hunter J O, 'Abnormal colonic fermentation in irritable bowel syndrome', **Lancet** (1998) 352; 1187-1189.

Hunter J O, 'Abnormal gut flora and food intolerance' in Brostoff J, and Challacombe S J, eds, **Food Allergy and Intolerance** (2nd edn), pp 343-50, Balliere Tindall, London, 2002.

Parker T J, Naylor S J, Riordan A M, and Hunter J O, 'Management of patients with food intolerance in irritable bowel syndrome: the development and use of an exclusion diet', **Journal of Human Nutrition and Dietetics** (1995) 8; 159-166.

CHAPTER 6

Atkinson R J, and Hunter J O, 'The Role of diet and of Bulking Agents in the Treatment of Irritable Bowel Syndrome' in Camilleri M, and Spiller R C, eds, **Irritable Bowel Syndrome diagnosis and treatment,** pp 141-150, W B Saunders, Edinburgh, 2002.

CHAPTER 7

Bradley D, **Hyperventilation Syndrome,** Kyle Cathie Ltd, London, 1998

Cluff, R A, 'Chronic Hyperventilation and its treatment by physiotherapy: discussion paper', **J Roy Soc Med** (1984) 77; 855-62

Han J N, Stegen K, De Valck C, Clement J, and Van de Woestinje K P, 'Influence of breathing therapy on complaints, anxiety and breathing pattern disorders in patients with hyperventilation syndrome and anxiety disorders', **J. Psychosom Res.** (1996) 41; 481-93

CHAPTER 8

Markwell S, **Constipation – lets get things moving,** Constable and Robinson, London, 2003.

Wald A, 'Constipation' in Bosch, Hawkey, and Weinstein, eds, **Clinical Gastroenterology and Hepatology; the modern clinician's guide,** Elsevier, Edinburgh, 2005.

CHAPTER 9

Bradley H K, Wyatt G M, Bayliss C E, and Hunter J O, 'Instability in the faecal flora of a patient suffering from food related irritable bowel syndrome', **Journal of Medical Microbiology** (1986) 22:1-4.

Hunter J O, Tuffnell Q, and Lee A J, 'Controlled Trial of Fructose-Oligosaccharide in the management of irritable bowel syndrome', **Journal of Nutrition** (1999) 129: 1451S-1453S

Sen S, Mullan M M, Parker T J, Woolner J T, Tarry S A, and Hunter J O, 'Effects of Lactobacillus plantarum 299v on Colonic Fermentation and symptoms of Irritable Bowel Syndrome', **Digestive Diseases and Sciences** 47, 2615-2620.

CHAPTER 11

Sparkes V, Prevost A T, and Hunter J O, 'Derivation and identification of questions that act as predictors of abdominal pain of musculo-skeletal origin', **Euro J Gastroenterol Hepatol** (2003) 15, 1021-7.

INDEX